Practical Radiance

30 Days to Brighter Living and Smarter Health

Trisha Bogucki, PharmD

Medical Disclaimer/Financial Disclosure

All material in this book is provided for informational or educational purposes only, and is not intended as a substitute for the advice provided by your healthcare professional or physician. Dr. Bogucki is a licensed pharmacist and makes several recommendations for products throughout the book. It is always best to consult your personal physician before trying any product. Please be sure to check all labels for allergy or sensitivity information. Dr. Bogucki hereby states that she has no relevant conflicts of inter est and no financial relationships or relationships to products or devices with any commercial interest. Only your physician knows your personal health history and can provide the treatment options appropriate for your specific condition. All efforts have been made to assure the accuracy of the information contained in this book as of the date of publication. Dr. Bogucki disclaims liability for any medical outcomes that may occur as a result of applying the methods or using the products suggested in this book.

Professional photography of Dr. Bogucki courtesy of Jenna Lynn Photography, South Jersey

ISBN: 0692919902
ISBN-13: 9780692919903

*Dedicated to the community and clients
that call me "pharmacist" - serving you is merely my job;
learning from you is my lifelong passion.*

*Thank you for giving this profession dimension,
significance, and purpose.*

CONTENTS

Trisha Bogucki

ACKNOWLEDGMENTS

To my husband and sons - in the words of Bryan Adams, "Everything I do, I do it for you." You're my world, my *joie de vivre*, and the reason for my laugh lines. Thank you for your constant love and support.

To my mom, Dolores Basu, whom I reference several times in this book - thank you for being my book editor and appointed life therapist. You and dad have given me so much in life. I only hope I've made you proud.

To my sister, Christina VanSkike - No matter how old we get and how much taller I am than you, I will always "look up to you." Thank you for your professional insight and the many years of sisterly giggles.

To the rest of my amazing family and in-laws - my appreciation only grows each day. Thank you for all you've done and continue to do to make life so worthwhile.

INTRODUCTION

JUST THE OTHER night I thought to myself, *Whatever higher power created the female probably didn't have her best interest in mind*. It wasn't the first time that this notion entered my subconscious, but I was still taken aback at myself. I always loved being a woman and embraced my femininity, even during my awkward years - and trust me, they were about as awkward as you can get. I have grown to know and appreciate all the qualities - both obvious and obscure - that separate us from our male counterparts and make all women beautiful in their own unique way. So why was I contemplating such a dismal thought? I was being facetious, of course, but couldn't help but think there was a teensy-weensy bit of truth to my theory that I was destined to live a tired life, plugging through the days on autopilot, and never truly feeling radiant. I'll elaborate more on where I was coming from at the time.

It was 4am, and the sound of babbling and "raspberries" was filling the void of what should've been a peaceful quietness. I hadn't had a decent night's sleep in months and was starting to think my five month old son had some sort of secret vendetta against those precious hours at night. I knew that in just a few hours, his brother - a highly energetic and precocious two year old - would come bounding down the stairs, ready to tackle the day with such a fierceness I was certain was inherited from their father. Once that moment came, there was no turning back on the day. I couldn't retreat to the cozy warmth of my bed no matter how exhausted I was. Work, bills, errands, and the insanely demanding task of caring for little children were lined up and not going anywhere anytime soon. Thank goodness I loved coffee!

My husband would be up in a few hours, too. He would complete his morning routine of getting breakfast and packing his bags for work. He is an amazing husband and father whose lifelong goal is to be there and take care of us. He doesn't frequent bars or demand "guy time" every single week. He is a great catch, and I'm glad we snagged each other at the ripe age of seventeen.

Even so, I thought about his life and day-to-day stresses. My husband exudes a quiet confidence that leads me to believe that his stresses don't drastically change over the years. Even on a purely physical level, he seems to age better with his mature looks becoming on him. Sure, he has his concerns about providing for his children, paying their college tuition, saving for retirement, and the like. These worries are enough to turn anyone's hair gray, and I would never try to minimize them. Plus, I'm certain he has other concerns that keep him up at night but doesn't feel the need to candidly share with me.

However, my husband conceals his stresses well and lives his life with the same ease he did a decade prior. Biologically speaking, he will never know the many discomforts of pregnancy or pain of childbirth. He can't understand why my mind is constantly running, worrying about seemingly silly concerns. He doesn't have a "biological clock" that sparks concerns if we ever decide to have more children. No, these are unique challenges that are distinctively "female," - albeit blessings disguised as hurdles.

I then turn my thoughts to my own parents. It was 4am - with no hopes of returning to bed anytime soon - so why not? My dad just turned seventy. He is Indian, so his dark skin coupled with silver hair give him a distinguished and sophisticated look. He made it through the ranks the hard way - growing up in poverty, learning English, and attending night school while working at an engineering firm during the day. He had some heart problems through the years, but he takes care of himself and lives for his grandchildren. He enjoys life with my mom - the strongest woman I know - by his side. She's the elegant matriarch that never really asked for much.

You would think my dad had it the hardest with coming to the States and trying a make a living, but it was actually my mom who bore the brunt of most of their difficulties. She was behind the scenes, dealing with the underlying pressures and stresses of raising three children with little money and an overworked husband. Much of what my dad initially earned went overseas to help support his relatives. Being that my mom is predominantly Irish-Catholic, cultural clashes often threatened the core of their marriage. But my mom was the unsung hero, the backbone of my dad's eventual success. To this day, she is acutely aware of all her grown children's needs and seems to experience the wonders of life's ups and downs a little more so than my dad.

From observing my mother, I've learned that the path of a woman's (and man's) life is akin to climbing a mountain with the stresses and demands of midlife coming in hard at the peak then tapering off as one grows closer to old age and retirement. Our bodies are built to handle life this way. Child rearing and hard work are meant for younger bodies that are resilient and capable of enduring the physical demands. As we age and our cells fight even harder to regenerate, life should seemingly slow down as well. Many folks in their seventies and eighties - if not riddled with too many physical ailments - still stay very active and enjoy a full schedule. But the incessant demands and "rat race" from yesteryears are a thing of the past, and most retirees are more than grateful for the slower pace.

Indeed, my mother would admit that the hardest part of her life was in her forties. I was an unplanned child - coming years after my brother and sister - so she still had me at home to look after in addition to caring for both her ailing mom and aunt. She often said this was a purgatory of sorts - a time when the care of the young matched the care of the old, and she thought she might crack under the constant demands of such extreme polarities. It was also during this time that she truly understood the brevity of life coming full circle. Even our family dog was growing old and required specialized attention. Many financial advisors agree that the forties and fifties are an important time to sock away for retirement, so the pressures of work and money were nagging at her too. Needless to say, she is relieved to be done with those years and enjoy the golden luster of retirement. She is also content to completely spoil her grandchildren but return them after a few hours of indulging their every demand. Thanks, mom.

Ok, so we know the female species are faced with a unique set of challenges that appear to cause all sorts of exhaustion and stress in our day-to-day lives. This is not new or groundbreaking news. I still had to ask myself if I - given my role as a modern woman - was destined to lead a lackluster life. Even my bleary eyes at 4am could see through the temptation to accept this notion. Because, in fact, the very elements and biological factors that contribute to our stress are also the same ones that help us to lead the most fulfilling and gratifying lives we possibly can. Let me explain by starting with the female brain.

While newer research suggests that the male and female brain are more alike than we think, it is still safe to say that we are hardwired a little differently from each other. The brain has four basic parts that control certain functions and are the same for both males and females.

We start with the brain stem which is the most primitive, controlling basic functions such as swallowing, balance, and our vital signs. We don't consciously think about these functions. The *limbic system*, or "reptilian brain," comes after the brain stem. The limbic system is responsible for our emotions, our "fight or flight" response, and pleasure center. It also houses the *basal ganglia*, which connects the limbic system to the more sophisticated *cerebral cortex*. The cerebral cortex is what separates us from other mammals. We develop language here, which helps us to make sense of the world and connect us to other human beings. Lastly, inside the cerebral cortex lies the *prefrontal cortex.* The prefrontal cortex is the final piece of the brain and takes the longest to fully mature, happening at around 19 to 24 years of age for most of us. It is the prefrontal cortex that allows us to have executive functioning. In other words, we learn the actions that contribute to a truly polished human being, such as expressing our emotions in a socially appropriate way, learning from our mistakes, and anticipating the consequences of our behavior. Undoubtedly, the prefrontal cortex is the most sophisticated piece of our brain and is really the "meat and potatoes" behind the decisions we make and the art of both forming and transforming habits. Ultimately, these habits and personal choices - though simple and overlooked - have the power to supersede our genetic predisposition to aging and disease. We are not destined for unhealthy living just because our genes make us susceptible.

The habits that we consistently do each and every day are the ultimate determinations of our health and radiance.

Despite the many similarities, the female brain is equipped slightly different from its male counterpart. Looking back in time, our prehistoric "sister's" main goal was to reproduce. Everything from fertilization to the nine months of growing a child and even to nourishing the young baby by breastfeeding was designed to take place in the female body. Because of this biological role, women have come to acquire a *mentalistic* mind - that in which we were meant to understand people in the most primitive of ways, such as nurturing a nonverbal infant or making allies in strange environments to ensure the safety of our offspring. Women are master empathizers - a quality that would ensure the survival of our prehistoric sister and her babies, but often seems to overwhelm us these days. *Am I a good enough mother? Am I doing enough for my children? Did I just say or do something to offend my friend, spouse, family member, etc?* These are all worries that stem from our unique ability to empathize - the quest to understand the emotions of other people and to be able to connect with them. We *want* to have good relationships and are constantly trying to be the best daughter, spouse, friend, worker, or mother we can be. And the result can be overwhelmingly stressful in our search for perfection. We pile too much on our plates in order to benefit everyone else in our lives, yet lose ourselves in the process. When was the last errand, chore, or duty you did that was strictly for *you?*

Yet - on a much more positive note - empathy is also why we can spark up conversations with other women in the grocery store, see when our spouses are stressed, and understand the needs of our children. Like I mentioned previously, my mother can still recognize when her adult children are stressed, even if we try to hide it with small talk or neighborhood gossip. She is the ultimate shoulder to lean on and shed a tear when we are beside ourselves. She understands that not all problems can be rationally or logically solved, but she will sure try. If she didn't have this capability, I truly believe her world would fall off its axis. When I think about how much my own loved ones need me, I realize that my world would suffer too if I lost this ability.

So yes, being a master empathizer can indeed be stressful. But our lives instantly become more radiant the minute we learn to take control of the pendulum and harness the ability to prioritize our personal needs as well. Revel in this dominant trait. Empathy makes the mind a formidable force by giving it dimension and substance. It strengthens the bonds we share with each other and is truly the most enriching and gratifying feature we could ever ask for in life.

Cognitive features aside, the female body is also laced with hormonal complexities that truly make us a work of biological art. You may not see this fact in such an optimistic light. You may think your hormones are the devil, contributing to body fat and giving you horrid PMS. This is true - a cascade of issues and health problems often ensue when our hormones become imbalanced. Overall, hormone levels gradually decline during the aging process, but imbalances and fluctuations naturally occur with puberty, pregnancy, and menopause. It is difficult to fight the hormonal pitfalls that Mother Nature bestowed upon us through these life events. But we can recognize the extrinsic factors that tend to lead our hormones astray, such as stress, toxins, and synthetic hormones in the form of medication. We can also recognize that our hormones are meant to be our "friends" and do wonderful things for our body. Estrogen - perhaps the most important female hormone - keeps our cholesterol under control, protects our bones, and is a key factor in determining our fertility.

When we evaluate just how special and beautiful our brain chemistry and bodies really are, we realize that every woman has the ability to lead a radiant life despite the many stresses and challenges that fall upon us. Keeping this in mind is difficult when life's demands are incessantly wearing us down. Many of us are over-caffeinated, over-medicated, and mentally overwhelmed with schedules and deadlines. The good news is that the struggle can be surmounted when we become cognizant of our needs, listen to our bodies, and make our health a priority.

Speaking of radiance, my personal definition means "lit from within." Good physical health is very easy to see on a cosmetic level. For instance, the whites around the eyes signify a good digestive system and the ability of the body to rid itself of toxins and wastes. Skin clarity and turgor indicate proper hydration and nourishment. Muscle tone means an active lifestyle in which our bodies are utilized for its strength and ability. However, to be "lit from within," the connections between mind and body must be nurtured and intact. We all know a certain someone in our lives who seems purely content and at peace with their world no matter how many struggles they face or flaws they have. "Lit from within" alludes to the constant process of bettering ourselves, our health, and vitality every day. It also means accepting the circumstances that we just cannot change. Feeling truly radiant on a cognitive level is happiness, confidence, and peace with the life we've made and the life that a higher power has planned for us. We learn to enjoy the journey and grow more each day. The learning process is never over, and perfection will never be achieved. In fact, I often feel that if we ever do reach a certain level of acceptance and complacency, then we're not really living life the way it's meant to be lived. The true radiant life will be speckled with flaws, but gratitude and a good sense of humor will help us to navigate the rocky roads and allow us to come out even better than before.

No amount of expensive beauty products will give us this type of radiance. Cosmetics, face creams, and costly procedures may give us an external boost, but will never adequately portray our inner glow. Almost anyone can tell if we're feeling tired, dull, or lifeless no matter how much mascara or blush we put on. Conversely, we truly radiate when we feel good, and it doesn't take much to shine. Such radiance is much more than physical.

I have to constantly remind myself that there is no such thing as perfection in beauty, and trying to keep up with celebrities or other superficially "beautiful" people can actually be detrimental to a woman's health. Being physically beautiful is not a worthy accomplishment if we are otherwise disengaged in the rest of life.

Yet when we eat well, stay active, live a little cleaner, and cultivate a peaceful and kind mind, we will begin to radiate a deep beauty that comes from within and is uniquely ours. And once we begin to see ourselves as radiant beings, we will naturally make better choices that nourish both our mind and body and help us live the best lives we can.

Life can be complicated and unpredictable. Injuries, illness, and disease can happen to even the most health-conscious person. Undoubtedly, we all will suffer from a prognosis sooner or later; some more complex and for longer periods than others. Such is the nature of the world we live in, and we must adapt to our circumstances the best way we can.

Fortunately, with the right treatments and lifestyle modifications, an overwhelming majority of ailments can be overcome or at least managed these days. Modern day medicine and alternative therapies can still afford a radiant life even with lifelong diagnoses, such as cardiovascular disease, diabetes, or epilepsy. More importantly, the human body is a beautiful and intricate system that is flexible, responsive, and self-healing. The mind and body should never be underestimated!

Aging gracefully

We need to recognize that our cells are continuously maturing and appreciate the value of the time we have. I worked as a clinical pharmacist for hospice patients for years. Most of the patients I worked with were elderly and had already accepted that death was imminent. Yet, some were young and had disease take them and their families by storm. Some were even babies - undoubtedly the saddest and most unfortunate of cases.

When faced with a terminal illness, people really evaluate the important things in life. Very rarely do people wish they made more money or had nicer things. *Time* is what people really want and can't get back - time spent with family and friends or time spent in peaceful solace.

The only way I know how to solve the problem of diminishing time is to actually sit down and log your day. Ask yourself these important questions to assess how well you are managing your time. *How much time is spent on commutes and lunch breaks? Can I possibly work from home or change my schedule to allow a more efficient work/life balance? How often do I check social media and get caught up in other people's lives? Are my children really benefiting from all of these activities? What are other things I can identify that are unnecessarily draining my time?*

When many people speak of aging gracefully, they mean it in a purely cosmetic sense - accepting the laugh lines, accentuating the silver streaks in hair, and avoiding Botox and fillers. To me, aging gracefully is a much more holistic phenomenon. It means embodying all aspects of the aging process, while taking care to not be negligent of the health we have now. Radiant health starts with our mind and heart. It starts with taking time for ourselves, being mindful of the choices we make, and fostering the important relationships we have. The physical part of radiant health will then follow.

A little about my philosophy

My background is pharmacy, having obtained my degree with a very Westernized approach to medicine. Western medicine relies heavily on *allopathy*, which means targeting the disease or symptom by using drugs or other remedies that cause the opposite effect. In fact, the term "allopathy" was coined by German physician, Samuel Hahnemann, and stems from the Greek *allos*, or "opposite", and *pathos*, or "suffering." Take the example of a runny nose. We usually administer an antihistamine - which causes a drying effect - to combat the symptom. The vast majority of drugs on the market exert this reversal of the body's mechanism.

Western medicine also strongly relies on "evidence-based" treatment, with results from clinical trials guiding doctor's drug choices and recommendations. I undoubtedly still believe in and make recommendations from proper evidence that something truly does work. However, my approach to healthcare is conceptually broad and holistic. I do not believe that drugs and chemicals are our first answer to all ailments, and I definitely don't adhere to a "one-size-fits-all" approach.

That's not to say I disparage Western medicine. I have seen many a family member in the hospital or suffer from conditions where pharmaceuticals are a must. The beauty of today's world is that we have access to proper medications to help us reach our optimal health, especially in the case of acute conditions or when other lifestyle modifications have failed. We shouldn't take for granted the cutting edge research and all of the options we have in today's healthcare.

What I do admonish, however, is medication misuse which can occur in many forms and is more common than you may think.

Overprescribing, polypharmacy (using multiple, unnecessary medications), and using other medications to treat side effects are all practices that abuse modern medicine and load our system with unnecessary chemicals.

Depending on the ailment, alternative medicine and lifestyle modifications should almost always be considered first over medication therapy. Countless studies have shown that non-drug therapy or a combination of such can be even more effective than popping a pill in many conditions, especially in chronic disease states that most likely didn't form overnight. Weighing the risks and benefits of such therapies is necessary, and a good practitioner will consider all aspects of treatment.

Balance really is key in life, and I am a firm believer that mental health goes hand-in-hand with our body's physical ability to function and perform. If our inner pendulum sways too harshly, our health and mental well-being may become suboptimal. For instance, it is very difficult to eat 100% organically or healthy all of the time, and I'd be a hypocrite to fully advocate such a diet. Afterall, I was born and raised in New Jersey - just outside of Philadelphia, to be exact - where a quality slice of pizza and glass of red wine can solve almost any problem! Conversely, we shouldn't be living on takeout and being sedentary every day either. A good life is one in which we practice healthy habits most of the time and try to live as "cleanly" as possible but also allow ourselves to live a little.

Health in Today's World

Many of us are already aware that medical information and advances are changing incessantly. With the advent of the internet and social media, we are inundated with a lot of different information, product endorsements, and societal opinions. I see it as a double-edge sword in most circumstances. Access to health information via the internet is convenient but so plentiful that many websites are inaccurate or even unnecessarily fear-provoking. It is extremely cumbersome to sift through the material to find a reputable source, even though our ability to procure such information is easier than ever before. Also, what is true and practiced now may not be in a few years or even months down the road. Living a balanced lifestyle that allows for some freedoms and choices helps to negate these continual changes and information overload. Practical knowledge, acceptance, and a good sense of humor go a long way in life.

Never underestimate the power of a woman's intuition when it comes to your health. Biology bestowed our intuition upon us long before it mattered how well-read or educated we were. Learn to listen to your body, become attuned to your hard-wirings, and not push yourself too hard in life.

The following guide contains pearls that are really meant to be tools in your toolbox. I've written them in no particular order, and they can be read at your leisure. Some are serious, whereas some are more lighthearted. The balance is indicative of what life should really be. I hope you find them to be as helpful in your life as they have been in mine.

Cheers to your radiance and mine,
Trisha Bogucki

30 DAY GUIDE TO BRIGHTER LIVING AND SMARTER HEALTH

Day 1
Adopt a fertile lifestyle

No matter what stage of life you're in or whether you choose to have children or not, any woman can benefit from the lifestyle changes that nurture and foster fertility and healthy womanhood. If bearing a child is on the horizon - but you'd like to hold off a little longer - you are definitely not alone! Motherhood is by far the most demanding "job" and perhaps you would like to finish your degree, establish a career, or do some traveling before parental demands kick in. Or, conversely, maybe you have already decided that children just aren't for you, but you could still benefit from a more vibrant lifestyle that allows you to feel fulfilled otherwise. If fertility is a concern for you, it is important to consider making a few minor - but important - changes before actively trying to conceive. Provided that half of all pregnancies are unplanned, it is probably a good idea to start paying more attention to these modifications if you're of childbearing age.

Most of the time, fertility is dependent upon two important factors - a male's sperm and a woman's egg. For men, how much sperm is produced, the quality of the sperm, and the mobility are the main issues that may prevent conception. For a woman, problems with ovulation are usually the major suspects. Without ovulation, there are simply no eggs to be fertilized.

Given this information, it is important to keep in mind the common "fertility busters" that could otherwise be damaging your health. Alcohol, caffeine, cigarette smoking, and recreational drugs have all been shown to negatively affect sperm count and ovulation. In fact, one major study found that when couples nixed these bad behaviors and took nutritional supplements, there was an eighty percent chance of conception.

Speaking of nutritional supplements, several have been purported to help women conceive. Even a relatively healthy diet can't provide all of the nutrients that are essential for both you and a potentially growing baby, so it's worth considering even if motherhood isn't in the near future. Luckily, a high quality prenatal vitamin contains most of these nutrients, such as folic acid; vitamins B-6, B-12, C, and E; magnesium; selenium; iron; and zinc. Another supplement that may help with fertility is the herb, vitex or chasteberry. Experts recommend taking 160-240mg daily for infertility. Good scientific data is lacking, but some research has indicated that the herb may be beneficial for women with luteal phase defects (shortened second half of the menstrual cycle). These women's ovaries generally don't produce enough progesterone. Chasteberry has been purported to normalize progesterone levels, which increases the chances of becoming pregnant.

Other lifestyle modifications to promote fertility include establishing regular patterns of sleep and exercise. Find a physician whom you like and trust, and make it a point to get yearly checkups for STDs and other health issues. Remember, even if a baby is the last thing on your mind, you still deserve to be in top health.

Most importantly, time is of the essence when it comes to fertility. There truly is never a "right" time to have a child - parenthood takes nearly everyone by storm, whether planned or not - so if you're on the fence, it may just be a matter of getting a few things in order and going for it while you still have youth, health, and energy on your side.

Prior to having children, I was at my gynecologist's office for a routine check-up when she inquired about potential motherhood. I was fiscally secure, had a home, and finished up secondary education - in other words, I was pretty much running out of "excuses" to keep putting it off. I knew I wanted to be a mother eventually, but something was always in the way. Maybe I could use another tropical vacation with my husband or put even more money away in the bank. When my doctor heard of my concerns, she said, "You're happy, healthy, and eventually want to be a mother - why not now?" It was her simplistic approach that cast my fears aside, and my husband and I started trying shortly thereafter. To this day, I'm thankful she was blunt with me. Of course, I could always use a vacation or more money. Anyone could. And of course, there is much to consider prior to having children. I would never advocate jumping the gun when it comes to motherhood. But waiting too long could be detrimental to your fertility. Being aware of this fact could save you heartache and the potential expense of costly fertility treatments down the road.

Day 2
Practice spirituality and mindfulness

It may come as a surprise, but spirituality is the number one predictor of longevity, good health, and happiness for both males and females. In case you find yourself shying away from the terminology, remember that being spiritual doesn't necessarily mean practicing an organized religion - it simply means having a system in place that allows you to reflect on the beauty of life and be able to find peace at any given moment. Try and find time to pray or meditate on a daily basis. If you initially feel uncomfortable, start simply by staring at a beautiful tree or body of water and practicing deep breathing exercises. Breathe from your stomach and diaphragm, as well as expand your entire chest and back. The act of deep breathing alone can stimulate the immune system, reduce stress, and bring oxygen into the body. Try not to complicate the process. Spirituality is whatever you need it to be to live a little more peacefully and healthfully.

Being mindful is another way to have truly radiant health. Mindfulness allows us to truly pay attention to our thoughts, actions, and senses at the present moment. If you feel like you are spending the majority of your life on "autopilot," you are probably not being very mindful. Mindfulness allows us to nurture the connections between a mental and physical state. So much of our physical health relies on a healthy mental outlook and being in a "right" state of mind. Undoubtedly, being mindful of the actions we take will have profound effects on our health and well-being. True and radiant health begins in the brain - we must *want* to have it, or else it will elude us.

When it comes to health, we can practice mindfulness in several ways. Renowned psychologist, Dr. Marsha Linehan, recommends remembering these three basic words to help you be mindful of any experience: *observe, describe,* and *participate.* Always be *observant* of the situation, taking note of not only your feelings and actions, but other people's as well. *Describe* your situation by putting words on the experience. Acknowledge each feeling and thought that enters your mind. Lastly, *participate* and get involved in your life. Put your cell phone away or stop trying to take the perfect picture. Cast worries aside and quit ruminating over the things you can't control. Your life is right here and right now, so jump in and be present.

Practice mindfulness while eating and exercising. Don't just pay attention to which foods you eat, but try to really savor and appreciate different tastes and textures. When you take the time to truly enjoy your food, it becomes harder to eat mindlessly while watching TV or doing work. When exercising, focus your mind on each muscle and ligament that's being worked. Breathe into your movements and stretches to make the most of them. Pay attention to your body and take heed when it feels "off". For women especially, our bodies and hormonal complexities sometimes have a funny way of telling us that something is wrong. For instance, heart attacks in women can present differently than heart attacks in men. Back or jaw pain and nausea or vomiting are often common symptoms in women. Being mindful of certain signs and symptoms - and not just brushing them off - could truly save lives.

Easy Yoga for Mindfulness

Yoga seems to be the "in" thing these days, as more and more people realize the benefits of a strong mind-body connection and an alternative way to ease the stress and tension of life's demands. Besides the physical benefits, yoga is a great way to incorporate mindfulness into your everyday life - often through breath awareness. People who practice yoga and other mindfulness techniques report being better able to deal with work issues, relationships, and other common stressors. Mindfulness simply gives you a better mental state and coping mechanism to help you deal with whatever issues lie ahead.

You don't have to be a "yogi" to do these simple exercises. You don't have to be young, hip, or sport the most fashionable yoga pants. These moves are easy, and you only need to take ten or fifteen minutes out of your day to reap the positive benefits.

Savasana

Lie on your back with your feet about a foot wide. Your arms should be at your sides with your palms up. Now, just focus on your breathing. Try to relax your breath and visualize it coming in and out. Don't let the day's worries or your to-do list infiltrate your mind as you breathe. If you do come across a thought, acknowledge it, and try to let it go as you continue to relax.

Cat-Cow Pose

I love doing this pose and will often take a couple quick minutes out of my day to sneak it in. I tend to hold a lot of tension in my back, and this is great way to stretch those muscles and relieve some of the discomfort. I also found this exercise to be my favorite while pregnant. Some experts even recommend cat-cow pose as a gentle way to get the baby in better position for birth.

Come on to your hands and knees, with your hands directly under your shoulders, and knees under your hips. Round your back as you exhale. Your tailbone should tilt between your legs. Rest your head forward so your eyes are looking at your thighs.

On the inhalation, bring your back down into a gentle backbend. Reach both your tailbone and head up towards the ceiling. You should feel a nice stretch and a little relief of any stiffness at this point. Continue to go back and forth between the "cat" and "cow" for a few times. Again, focus your breathing as you do the moves, and try not to let your mind wander.

Downward-Facing Dog

From the cat-cow pose, tuck your toes, lift your hips, and straighten your legs. You are now in downward-facing dog pose. Try and hold this position with your legs straightened for about 10 breaths. This is another great exercise to stretch the back, legs, and hamstrings. Try pumping your heels up and down for an added stretch.

Tadasana (Mountain Pose)

Stand with your feet firmly on the ground and arms at your sides. Try to distribute your body weight evenly, relax your shoulders, and keep your chin parallel to the floor. Ease any tension you may be carrying in any muscle. Picture yourself as a mountain - grounded and calm.

Day 3
Be the ultimate keeper of your home

A dark, cluttered, and disorganized home often speaks more of the owner than it does of the physical space. Make every effort to keep your living space comfortable, reflective of your personal style, and welcoming to guests. Fresh flowers, scented candles, and a few well-appointed decorative items can go a long way.

Take pride in your home and revel in the simple pleasures that make your space unique. Perhaps you love a signature fragrance or maybe collect beautiful tabletop linens. Both your guests and your children will appreciate these nuances and remember them for years to come. An example would be my parent's home - a space so modest that I sometimes wonder how they raised three children in those walls. Yet, my mom absolutely adores her home, and has always loved elegant decor even when we kids were little and acted like the proverbial "bulls in a china shop". She would adorn every tabletop with pictures in beautiful, yet mismatched frames and take the time to fold cloth napkins in fancy rings when entertaining. Now that she's retired and is an empty-nester, her new splurges are with the designer, Mackenzie Childs. The checkered pattern looks so sophisticated and literally right at home in her dining room and kitchen. It is a true pleasure to visit my childhood home and see my mom's signature style, and I can only hope that my own children appreciate the care and energy I put into our own to make it happy and special.

Another tip would be to invest in what I call "functional furniture" - furniture with hidden storage compartments or organizational pieces that can help keep paperwork, kid's toys, and other clutter at bay. After my first son was born, the encroachment of his "stuff" in our living space was surprisingly overwhelming me. I instantly bought a plush storage bench with plenty of room for his toys and books and two end tables with compartments to hide his diapers and wipes. They were the best furniture investments I ever made. Needless to say, your home should be bright, warm, comfortable, and free of too much clutter. Even the smallest of apartments can be made into your personal sanctuary with the right outlook.

Try to use non-toxic cleaners for your home as much as possible. Many commercially available cleaners are chock full of toxins, harsh chemicals, and even pesticides. These ingredients can contribute to cancer, asthma, and other respiratory diseases. Don't let your home become a danger zone to yourself and your little ones. My favorite cleaner is something I concoct myself and couldn't be more simple:

1 cup water

1 cup vinegar

roughly 40 drops of lemon, clove, or tea tree oil

These oils have germ-fighting qualities and really cut through the vinegar scent. I frequently use baby wipes as well. If they are sensitive enough for my baby's bottom, then I can be sure they won't harm my granite countertops or wooden kitchen table. And one of my favorite ways to make my kitchen sink sparkle is to sprinkle baking soda and then scrub with the flat part of half a lemon.

Certain places and items around the home can be hard to clean using a homemade concoction. If I ever use a commercial product, I try to make sure it is as plant-based as possible. For instance, I rely on a brand called Therapy for my stainless steel appliances, which is coconut oil - based. I only use bleach or other harsh chemicals if I absolutely have to - for example, if I've been working sloppily with raw meats on the counter, one of my children has a major accident somewhere, or if a pretty bad illness is running through my family. My mom somehow contracted a bad case of salmonella last year, so I've seen firsthand how debilitating that can be. I'm very particular about keeping the counters clean after working with raw meats. You have to weigh the risks and benefits of when to use harsher chemicals.

The Fifteen Minute Clean-Up

Many household connoisseurs recommend "the fifteen minute clean-up." I first read of this in Jennifer Scott's, "At Home with Madame Chic: Becoming a Connoisseur of Daily Life." It simply means setting your kitchen timer for fifteen minutes and doing as much as you can during that time. I will be the first to admit that by the end of the day, I'm spent. It often takes the last of my energy reserves to just put the kids to bed. But when I commit to these fifteen minutes, I surprise myself with how much I can truly accomplish. And waking up to somewhat presentable house the next morning is a great way to start the day. Plus, on an even better note, it saves me from spending a couple of hours cleaning the home on those precious weekends. Doing a little at a time makes the mundane task of cleaning a little more palatable and actually saves you more time and energy in the long run.

Day 4
Entertain and be entertained...

Humans, by nature, are social creatures. Face-to-face interaction - not text, email, or even phone calls - is essential to our health! While not all of us are blessed with Paris Hilton's social life (or have the time, energy, or money for one), we should try to make the most of entertaining and social events when the opportunities arise. Engage in conversation, make eye contact, and smile warmly. Make it a point to show interest and truly listen to people when they talk. Yet, know when to elegantly excuse yourself with the promise of catching up later if situations or conversations turn awkward.

Brush up on some basic etiquette whenever guests come over - even unexpectedly - such as always offering food or drink and making sure they are comfortable. A glowing hostess always puts their guests first and doesn't truly relax until everyone else has. Conversely, if you're attending someone else's event, it should go without saying to never show up empty handed. To avoid being a total clod in the social department, try to always keep on hand a few bottles of wine (for both offering guests and for giving as gifts), classy thank you notes and other greeting cards, and a few decent-quality serveware items. By cultivating a sense of community and social interaction, you will help keep your brain and mind healthy as you age.

Day 5
...but know when to say "No"

Respectfully declining requests or other opportunities when your plate is already full does not make you a bad person. It simply means you've evaluated your priorities and recognized that not everything is worth your time and energy.

I still find it difficult to say "no" sometimes. I have been and will always naturally be a "yes" girl. I feel as though I am destined for this attribute. I was the "baby" of the family growing up, and I'm used to older siblings calling the shots and going along with it.

Or, perhaps, maybe it is because I am a Pisces. Pisceans are known for going with the flow and keeping the peace. Whatever the reason may be for my placating, I have always found it easier in life to just say "yes."

But that was when I was younger and naive. These days, I have a job, marriage, a home, children, and a high-maintenance diva of a Pomeranian all needing exorbitant amounts of my attention. If you're reading this, no doubt you have your own list of people and things that require your care. So maybe I can safely assume that you sometimes feel like a waitress at a fancy restaurant with a bunch of items on their serving tray. This is how I feel on most days too, and I know everything will fall if I am not careful. This juggling act is often why I remind myself to always be cognizant of what's on my tray and to never overload it. We need to balance our time and energy and conserve them for those we love and who truly need us. This means getting used to - and not feeling bad about - saying "no" to other recipients deemed unworthy from time to time.

Day 6
Ask for help

Outsource to a practical degree. A lot of women tend to bite off more than they can chew. Believe me when I say that stress is a silent killer. It will deplete you of your health and radiance and put you at risk for a host of health issues. Back when I was a young intern, the successful owner of the pharmacy I was working for gave me some sage advice. He said that a good pharmacist knows how to do every single thing in the pharmacy, but a great pharmacist delegates the tasks that overload his time and energy. I often remember that advice as matriarch of the household. Even if temporarily, consider hiring a housecleaner, a regular sitter for the kids for a couple of hours, or other forms of help with food shopping and errands. If you're having trouble justifying the cost of outsourcing, consider seeking assistance from a cash-strapped college or high school student or perhaps someone you know that has just lost their job and is looking for side work. It's a two-way street, and you may just be helping them more.

Day 7
Get out of debt

Many women don't realize how much of a burden debt really is until it has been lifted from their shoulders. Financial stress will put more wrinkles on your face than age itself. Money problems are still the leading cause of failed marriages and why so many college graduates are still living out of their parents' basement. If your spouse prefers to handle the finances, don't use this as an excuse to bury your head in the sand. Always know what's coming in and what's going out - it is the only way to ever overcome debt. Find out exactly where your money is going and avoid hidden fees and surcharges that are attached to almost every service these days. If you have to enlist the help of a trustworthy financial advisor, do so.

Maybe you happen to be debt-free. If so, start investing in ways that can make your money work for you. Look for other modes of income and don't rely too heavily on your main job to give you financial freedom. The extra cash coming in from smart investments or side work will help you sleep better at night and ease unnecessary tension in your relationships. Don't be afraid of money. After all, power is the root of all evil, not money.

Day 8
Write things down

Everything from doctor's appointments, deadlines, birthdays, and even your hopes and dreams - write it down or electronically log it. Don't let these important events or tasks escape to the nether regions of your brain, only to be remembered in the middle of the night or while driving to work. Staying organized will do wonders for your life and save you time and energy in the long run. Research has also shown that even writing down your aspirations can help you better achieve them.

Check your calendar often and always be aware of the type of day/week you're up against. I'm a very visual person, so if I see that I have a lot going on in my calendar during a particular time, I am better able to prepare myself both mentally and physically and do things ahead of time to space out my load.

Therapeutic Journaling

Writing can help us find mental peace, too. One of the most enlightening seminars I've ever attended was conducted by Dr. Joseph Shannon and entitled "Changing How We Feel by Changing How We Think." Our mindsets are such an important factor in determining our health and how we live. He recommends therapeutic journaling as a way to overcome traumatic life events and change problematic mindsets that prevent us from living life fully. The guidelines are as follows:

1. Write in a private place where you will not be distracted or interrupted .

2. Focus on the traumatic experiences in your life, and be sure to include the details that are most difficult to acknowledge.

3. As you write, shift your focus from external events to the internal thoughts and feelings you experienced in response to those events.

4. Write for around twenty minutes per day for at least four consecutive days. Don't worry about grammar or syntax. Writing repeatedly about the same experience may help improve your clarity and feelings about the event.

5. After you have written, think about how you can transform this painful experience into something positive. What aspects about the event have given you substance, clarity, insight, or wisdom?

6. Share your story with a safe, supportive individual.

7. Schedule a transitional activity - such as prayer or music therapy - to return to life as usual.

Day 9
Treat your inner circle like gold

Finding friends that are trustworthy, inspirational, and sincere is a tough task these days. However, life is too hectic to have a million fair weather friends - people that seem to hang around when it suits them or pretend to be interested in the details of your life only if such knowledge is advantageous to them. Try to be courteous to everyone, but start prioritizing the people in your life that are worthy of your attention.

If you do manage to cultivate a strong inner circle of family and/or friends, consider yourself fortunate and treat them kindly. Respond timely to correspondences, and make sure they know how important the relationship means to you. Having a positive support system can help you navigate through the tough times and make the good times that much better.

Day 10
Treat your spouse/significant other like gold, too

Your marriage will most likely (and hopefully) still be there long after the kids have grown, you have retired, and the house has been sold in favor of a one story rancher in Florida. Ok, this may not be your exact situation, but you get my point! Hopefully, your life partner can be the one constant when everything else changes. Be honest, considerate, and put them first. Don't wait until the divorce papers have been signed or relationship ended to change your hair, lose weight, and smile more. And definitely don't treat your boss or outsiders nicer than your spouse.

You may find that many of your spousal arguments happen at night after a long day of work for the both of you. Stresses on the job can seep into household affairs, and it is important to not take the day's events out on your spouse. I've seen this happen with my own parents, and it happens with my marriage, too. If this is the case for you, try doing something stress-relieving immediately after work like going for a walk or to the gym, or even just grabbing a cup of coffee and reading the newspaper by yourself. You're likely to be in a better mood when you arrive home and are in better position to ward off unnecessary bickering or nitpicking. Your better mood might rub off on your spouse, too.

Look, I know humans are capable of doing awful things. I also recognize that some problems have run too deep and for too long to be solved. In fact, research has indicated that staying in an unhealthy or abusive relationship can shave between ten and fifteen years off of your life expectancy! I can't be the judge of your particular situation, and I won't pretend that cooking a nice meal or surprising your loved one with a weekend getaway will eradicate profound issues. But I do know a lot of good can happen when we consistently and unequivocally bring our best to the relationship and keep on top of notorious perpetrators.

Day 11
Differentiate between good and bad advice

Back when I became pregnant for the first time, it seemed as if every mother had a word of advice to offer about all things childcare and parenthood. I'm always amenable to receiving words of wisdom, but the onslaught of opinions was frustrating at times. Trust yourself to recognize the helpful advice in life. I learned the hard way that no one really intends to be ill-willed, but maybe just isn't aware of all the details to have your best interest in mind. A classy woman will be outwardly polite and consider everything, but inwardly absorb only what's good for her.

Day 12
Practice Kegel exercises daily

Many women suffer from annoying and sometimes even painful "pelvic floor" issues, such as an incontinent bladder. Whether you have had children or not, it is important to remember that the pelvic floor is indeed a muscle that needs attention and strengthening just like any other muscle in the body.

In France, their national health service often prescribes and will even cover the expenses of pelvic floor strengthening after childbirth.

This rehabilitation program is usually a series of sessions that include physical therapy to help restore strength to the weakened pelvic floor after the trauma of pregnancy and delivery. Often given just weeks after birth, such attention to those private muscles helps to prevent leaky bladder, pelvic pain, and pelvic organ prolapse.

I believe we are a bit lagging in the States when it comes to this realm. Undisputedly, we have top-notch prenatal care and even pediatric care for the child once he or she is born. Yet, we are often left to our own devices when it comes to postpartum health. Given that nearly 50 percent of all women suffer with urinary leakage and 25 percent with pelvic prolapse, every woman - regardless of childbirth - should be well educated on how to strengthen her pelvic floor. I believe training should start from the very first gynecological appointment as teenagers.

Aim to do at least 50 Kegel exercises a day. Imagine you are trying to stop urinating, and contract that muscle. If you can, try practicing Kegels in a squatting or lunging position. The added lengthening of the pelvic floor will make them even more effective.

Day 13
Cultivate a proper skincare regimen

One of the most obvious ways to show your radiance is to have healthy, glowing skin. Given that your skin is the body's largest organ, it's important to take of it from both the outside as well as from the inside. Your skin can be a great indicator of a lot of your daily habits. This can be a good thing or a bad thing! Genes and environmental factors play major roles in skin health, so don't despair if you've been neglectful. In fact, it's never too late to start a good skincare regimen. Most, if not all, dermatologists will stress prevention and the importance of keeping up with the basics.

There was a time not long ago when I could indulge in a few cocktails until the wee hours of the morning and still manage to make it to an 8am class looking (and even feeling!) like a million bucks. Alcohol, sleep deprivation, and processed breakfast sandwiches on the run just didn't seem to affect the outwardly appearance of my skin during this highly coveted part of my youth. I was in my early twenties and had that youthful glow that so many "older" folk break the bank to recapture.

I don't have to tell you that it's a different story these days. Let's just say that it's a little too easy to look lackluster. I love my professional camera that my husband bought for me as a gift, but hate that the pictures are detailed enough to showcase crow's feet, sunspots, dark undereye circles, and enlarged pores. Skin is one of the body's first line of defense to just about everything. And given all that mine has been exposed to over the years, it's no wonder that imperfections have surfaced.

Whole textbooks exist on skincare and an overabundance of products line the shelves, but you really only need to adopt some basic practices and be aware of some of the common offenders that can deplete your skin of its radiance. One thing I can stress is that most of the time, it really doesn't matter which product you decide to use or how much it costs - just the act of keeping up with a regimen on a consistent basis is enough to keep it healthy and glowing.

First things first - you absolutely, positively need to wear sunscreen. Your mother may have been on to something when she chided you for not protecting yourself. Rain or shine, hot or cold - ALWAYS wear an SPF. The sun is one of the biggest culprits of aging skin and can be responsible for fine lines, sunspots, and dangerous skin cancers. I like to recommend sunscreen that contains physical - as opposed to chemical - sun blockers. These ingredients are usually zinc oxide or titanium dioxide and are safe enough to be found in baby sunscreen. If you're looking for an "adult" version, I recommend the brand, Coola. Coola's other ingredients are usually plant-based and organic, so it really is a safe bet when it comes to skincare. I especially like their mineral BB cream. If wearing sunscreen under makeup, apply it and then do something else, like brush your teeth or style your hair. The extra few minutes will allow your skin to absorb the sunscreen and not be rubbed away by makeup.

Most people don't wear enough sunscreen, or many feel that an SPF-containing foundation is enough for proper protection. Remember that SPF ratings are determined in an laboratory environment, where conditions are prime and the testers are not moving or sweating. Laboratory environments are rarely indicative of real life, so we have to be mindful of all the confounding factors that make an SPF less effective for the common individual. Use at least a teaspoonful of sunscreen for just your face, and reapply it every couple of hours if you're very active or swimming. Don't forget to apply it to your neck and chest, as well.

The American Academy of Dermatology recommends wearing an SPF of at least 30, which will block 97 percent of the sun's rays. Look for a sunscreen that provides both UVA and UVB coverage. Try to be amenable to physical blockade if you tend to be forgetful with applying an SPF. Broad-rimmed hats and long-sleeves are also great ways to block out harmful rays. Even though it is sometimes difficult, I try to schedule beach days - or other times when my family and I will be exposed to a lot of sun - during the early morning hours or after 3:00 p.m., when the sun's rays are less strong. Another added benefit is the lack of crowds during these times.

Exfoliation is another key to success when it comes to skincare. Men often look younger than woman, purportedly due to the daily facial shaving that removes dead skin cells and allows new ones to resurface. Exfoliation can be done either mechanically or chemically, and it really all depends on your skin type. Those with sensitive skin should use a mild mechanical exfoliant, such as jojoba beads, and limit their exfoliation to a few times a month. Whereas those with thicker, oily skin can get away with a stronger chemical or mechanical exfoliation, such as a brush or a scrub. Examples of stronger chemical exfoliants include lactic acid or glycolic acid.

Exfoliation can dry out the skin and should be done cautiously if skin is being treated with acne medication, which are often retinoid-containing products or benzoyl peroxide. No matter your skin type or how often you exfoliate, a moisturizer should always be applied afterwards to prevent dryness.

Microdermabrasion is another way to exfoliate the skin by gently "sanding" away the outer layer. This is usually done at a medical spa, but some products are available for at-home use. On the very rare occasion that I actually treat myself to a facial at a spa, I like to add microdermabrasion on as a way to rejuvenate my skin and smooth out the texture. This is another great preventative way to avoid some of the harsher, artificial skin procedures.

The final key to success when it comes to skincare is proper moisturizing. Use an antioxidant-rich moisturizer daily and start as soon as you can. I like moisturizers that contain any or all of the following antioxidants: vitamin C, vitamin E, resveratrol, green tea, and retinol. Applying moisturizer on a daily basis embodies two major components of aging naturally: preservation and prevention.

A Sample Skin Care Regimen:

Morning

Wash face with a creamy, mild cleanser. *Examples: Dove, Cetaphil*

Apply an antioxidant-rich moisturizer with an SPF of 30. *Examples: Coola SPF 30 Face Classic Sunscreen, Aveeno Positively Radiant Daily Facial Moisturizer*

Evening

Wash face. You could even do a "waterless" washing using micellar water or makeup wipes. If using the waterless way, be sure to properly remove any lipstick or eye makeup using another product, if necessary. *Examples: Simple Micellar Cleansing Water, Lancome Bi-Facil Double Action Eye Makeup Remover*

Use a toner to deeply cleanse. Examples: *Avalon Organics Vitamin C Facial Toner, Pixi Glow Tonic*

Apply a facial serum or oil. *Examples: Caudalie Radiance Serum, Palmer's Facial Oil*

Apply a nighttime moisturizer. *Examples: Yes to Coconut Overnight Creme, Origins Night-a-Mins*

Gently dab on undereye cream. *Examples: Neutrogena Rapid Wrinkle Repair Eye Cream, Estee Lauder Advanced Eye Cream*

Twice a Week

Exfoliate skin to remove dead cells and allow new ones to surface. *Examples: Burt's Bees Citrus Facial Scrub, Vasanti Enzymatic Face Rejuvenator*

Apply a facial mask. *Examples: I like to make my own using a variety of fresh ingredients such as Greek yogurt, honey, avocado, egg whites, organic coconut oil or fresh lemon juice. I never use a particular recipe and just mix ingredients together until the consistency is right.*

Once a Month

I recommend using a gentle, at-home microneedling system. My husband saw my inexpensive microneedling system that I purchased from Amazon and thought it looked like a miniature medieval torture device. I won't lie - it looks weird, sounds weird, and even feels a little weird. But the grounds for microneedling is actually very primitive in nature and can be a great preventative way to stay out of the doctor's office for expensive and sometimes even dangerous facial procedures.

Microneedling uses very small needles to gently prick the skin. The body senses these tiny injuries and triggers collagen and elastin production to heal. The result can be improved texture and skin tone, as well a reduction in stretch marks or scars. In fact, I have found microneedling to be one of the only ways to reduce my stomach stretch marks from pregnancy.

The best way to use a microneedling device is to gently roll several times in different directions on clean, dry skin. I like to do this at night, right before I apply a mild nighttime lotion in order to aid the absorption. Be careful to use only gentle products afterwards, and refrain from using cosmetics, sunscreen, facial "peels", or other harsh ingredients. If you decide to try microneedling, take care to use a very small needle - about 0.5 millimeters - and use a gentle touch. Be sure to keep your microneedling device clean with warm, soapy water. I recommend using a microneedling device only once a month, as this is a fairly new and novel procedure and essentially creates a thicker skin. You definitely don't want to overdo it.

Healthy Skin, Hair, and, Nails From the Inside Out - Collagen 101

By far, the best supplement that I've invested in on a purely superficial level has been collagen. That's because skin, hair, and nail health aside, collagen is actually rich in antioxidants and has positive effects on many important functions of the body. Benefits include:

Stronger bones, ligaments, and tendons
Stronger connective tissue for better mobility and elasticity
Better circulation
Potentially lower blood pressure

Collagen is actually the most abundant protein in the human body and is very well absorbed in the blood stream after oral consumption, so you can be certain that a high-quality collagen supplement is doing its job.

As we age, our body's production of collagen starts to slow down. In fact, breakdown will actually exceed production leading to wrinkles, weak fingernails, and saggy skin. Low collagen levels can even lead to weak teeth, bones, and connective tissues.

Supplementing with straight collagen or bone broth, which is incredibly high in collagen, is a great way to overcome this natural process and help keep us glowing and strong.

Bone broth is very easy to procure or even make yourself by submerging chicken bones in water in a slow cooker. Drinking a warm cup everyday is a great way to help stave off the aging process. If you feel that bone broth is not for you, look for a high-quality supplement. I use a product called Neocell, which is available as either a powder for mixing or a pill. Neocell is absorbed nicely and uses food grade collagen.

Day 14
Get a good night's sleep

Beautiful Hollywood actress Heather Graham swears by getting at least 10 hours of sleep every night. She knows it sounds excessive to some people, but she can't imagine sleeping any less. She is forty-seven years old and can easily pass for at least a decade younger, exuding a natural radiance that seems to be a rarity on the artificially-enhanced red carpet these days. So is sleep really the fountain of youth?

Sleep is more beneficial than many of us realize and is critical for radiant, vibrant health. Adequate sleep strengthens our immune function and metabolism and also helps in memory, learning, and other vital processes. We also look better when we are well-rested and are able to let our bodies heal at night. Adequate sleep - consisting of around eight hours per night - seems like such a simple remedy for so many health problems, but roughly thirty percent of Americans get six hours of sleep or less. In essence, we lead fast-paced lives with grueling schedules. Stress, caffeine, and a world abuzz with electronic devices all keep us going well into the evening hours. We may seem to function well enough for a while, but sleep deprivation will eventually affect our core, altering hormone levels, gene function, and even life expectancy.

You may be a new mom or a mom to young children and think to yourself, *Sure, sleep is great - if I could get some.* Or maybe you've been afflicted with another condition that prevents a good night's sleep. I know plenty of women with urinary incontinence, restless leg syndrome, anxiety about current events, or other symptoms that affect sleep quality. I'm no stranger to stone cold exhaustion and know that sleep becomes a hot commodity the minute it's been robbed from me.

If you do happen to be a new mom, the only words of encouragement I can offer is that babies don't keep, and neither do their tortuous sleep schedules. No matter the habits or personality, it is a child's natural inclination to begin sleeping through the night at some point. They will sleep, and so will you - eventually. In the meantime, you will have to slow down other aspects of your life to account for the lack of sleep and constant physical and emotional energy that caring for young children requires. I didn't realize this notion with my first baby, and I ended up paying the price.

My first son was only five months old at the time, but I had already been back to work for months and simultaneously doing some renovation on my home. My husband was turning thirty during all of this, and it was my ultimate goal to give him a big, fancy party at our house. It was a lot on my plate as a first time mom, and I thought I'd be failing if I couldn't handle it all.

The day before the party, I was running around like a mad woman trying to get everything in order. I wanted every detail and nuance to be perfect. Everything from the bartender to the three-tier cake was all finalized and ready to go for the next day.

As I slept in bed that night, I felt that something was physically "off" with me. As soon as I got up to use the bathroom, I collapsed like a sack of potatoes, shattering the bridge of my nose on the edge of one of the bathroom tiles. I somehow came to my senses, got up, and fainted yet again next to the bed! My husband heard me fall this time and came to my rescue. It was only with the help of ice, ibuprofen, and massive amounts of concealer that I was able to get through the next day relatively unscathed.

The following Monday, I saw my doctor for a full checkup and nose evaluation. He confirmed that I had indeed broke my nose, with the only culprit for my blackouts being pure exhaustion.

Lack of sleep associated with motherhood is a natural rite of passage that, unfortunately, must be accepted to some degree. However, it is impossible to maintain a full schedule during the day if you're not making up for the energy loss at night. You may even find yourself having to physically slow your pace when it comes to running errands or completing household chores. Remember, it takes a full year for your body to heal from childbirth. Special care needs to be taken during this time to nourish yourself and replenish your nutrient stores. As with many other situations in life, keep in mind that this point in time is temporary. You will feel like yourself again and be able to resume your fun, action-packed life - only with a bouncing child in tow!

Sleep should always try to be attained as naturally as possible to allow for a deep, restorative state. Some methods include, but are not limited to the following:

Try to keep sleep and wake times consistent every day. Ayurvedic medicine suggests a routine of going to bed at approximately 10:00 p.m. and arising at approximately 6:00 a.m. Hormones that heal the body are released between 10:00 p.m. and 2:00 a.m., and are only released when the body is in a deep sleep.

Treat unresolved issues that are making sleep difficult, such as injuries, sleep apnea, or other illnesses.

Stay active during the day with plenty of activity and fresh air.

Omit caffeine and alcohol after 3pm, or even earlier if you are sensitive to the effects of either substance.

Keep your bed for sleep only. Don't read, watch TV, work, worry, or discuss problems in bed.

Avoid the use of cell phones and laptops in bed. The blue light emitted from technological devices suppresses the production of melatonin, the hormone that controls the sleep/wake cycle. These devices keep our minds alert and distract us during the night.

Give yourself a half hour to unwind before bed. Do something relaxing, such as a hot bath or shower.

Keep your room as comfortable as possible. Invest in a good mattress and bedding. Use pillows that adequately support your head and neck.

Use alarms with gentle tones that ease the body out of sleep and don't shock the system first thing in the morning.

Try an herbal tea that contains relaxing compounds, such as chamomile or valerian root.

Short-term use of melatonin, a hormone that aids in the sleep-wake cycle, can help in situations like jet lag, shift work, or other situations where sleep doesn't come naturally.

The Hidden Dangers of Sleep Aids

Both over-the-counter and prescription sleep aids are widely used and misused. Disruptions in sleep - whether it be difficulty in falling asleep, staying asleep, or both - is a often a transient phenomenon related to a life event or perhaps another untreated diagnosis. In the long run, sleeping pills are unlikely to help insomnia and may actually do more harm than good.

Some side effects of sleep aids include a next morning "hangover", feeling dizzy or lethargic the following day, memory loss, and difficulty concentrating. Most sleep aids can actually prevent your body from getting into a deep sleep - a sleep that is absolutely critical for repair, restoration, and truly vibrant health. This artificially induced "zone" can lead to sleepwalking or other abnormal sleep-related behaviors. Some evidence shows that long term use of sleep aids may even lead to dementia and brain damage, and this notion is most likely attributable to the aforementioned "fake" sleep. The brain is never getting to a point at night where the cells can repair and recharge.

Sleep aids induce an artificial sleep which doesn't allow the brain and body to fully heal at night.

Many over-the-counter sleep products are actually antihistamines, which have a drying effect on the whole body. Yet, prescription sleep aids are not any safer, even those that are shorter acting or have different purported mechanisms of action. A host of data tells us that women and older people are extra sensitive to the side effects of all sleep aids, especially prescription ones. And when mixed with alcohol or other medications such as pain relievers or antianxiety medications, the potential for dangerous side effects multiplies exponentially. Perhaps the biggest concern is the high potential to become dependent on them. Many people report having "rebound" problems with sleep or withdrawal side effects if they stop using them.

On any given day, an unbelievable amount of people are driving, working, and otherwise "functioning" with sleep aids still in their system. The secondary effects of possible car accidents and work mishaps can be even scarier and need to be considered as well. So what do we do when the occasional illness, injury, or life event occurs that prevents us from attaining sleep which is so critical for radiant health? Judicious use of sleep aids for one or two weeks probably won't present too much of a risk. Use the lowest dose possible and avoid taking it with any other medications that depress the system. Be careful with cough and cold products as well, as many contain antihistamines which cause further drowsiness. If you're still having problems with sleep after a couple of weeks, start paying attention to other behaviors or untreated illnesses that could be contributing to the issue. Behavioral therapy and good sleep habits are actually the best ways to treat sleep problems long term.

Day 15
Reduce electromagnetic chaos as much as possible

Evidence exists that electromagnetic waves can, to some degree, cause a myriad of health issues and cancers. This is a hard one, because electromagnetic waves are literally everywhere. We can't avoid them or eliminate them completely, but we can be a little more proactive in our daily routines. Never sleep next to a charging cell phone. Not only will keeping your cell phone far away from you at night reduce the emitting waves, it will also reduce your temptation to constantly check it.

Try to reduce the amount of food you microwave and avoid microwaving in plastics as much as you can. Toxic chemicals from plastic can leak out into food when heated. Resisting the urge to "steam" vegetables in plastic bags or heat up leftovers in plastic storage containers is hard, but a much safer option. This is particularly difficult for me and probably the majority of busy moms, as it almost always involves having to clean another dish.

And lastly, aside from the more obvious reasons, lessen your time watching TV.

Day 16
Pay attention to foot health

We don't give our feet nearly as much attention as we should. If you're like me and just can't resist a gorgeous heel from time to time, use a gel or padded insert to help alleviate foot pain and promote strong arches. The vast majority of us use and abuse our feet daily with physical activity and ill-fitting shoes, but they deserve much more than that. Our feet connect us to the earth and literally keep us grounded. Ancient healing traditions in China and India recognize that proper foot health represents overall wellbeing. Foot ailments can be indicative of other more serious conditions - such as diabetes and arthritis - and can even propagate to leg, neck, and back pain. I can't tell you how many times my whole body seemed to feel sore after a night out wearing high-heeled, uncomfortable shoes. In fact, Israeli actress Gal Gadot eschewed fancy stilettos in favor of comfortable flats for her red carpet appearances promoting the movie "Wonder Woman." Her practical reasoning? She stated that stilettos put you off-balance and give you back pain. No one has to remind me of that!

If you have a job that requires you to spend hours on your feet each day, promoting good foot health applies even more to you. Make sure to wear comfortable shoes and/or orthotics and give your feet a break from time to time. Find footwear that supports your arch and fits well. Even if you work in a environment that adulates heels, don't let fancy shoes give you bad feet!

Day 17
Put the drink down

I won't lie. Sometimes the sound of a good quality wine being poured into a glass is like music to my ears after a long, stressful day. I love the occasional alcoholic beverage, and there is never a shortage of options for our guests when we entertain or host large parties. In fact, I just came across a recipe for a "Hawaiian Mimosa" - which contains coconut rum, pineapple juice, and champagne, for those that are interested - and I can't wait for our next brunch or special occasion to try this fancy cocktail.

There is nothing wrong with a nightly glass of red wine with dinner (or other occasional beverage). Red wine actually has a plentitude of health benefits and has been purported to be the reason behind the Mediterranean and Eastern European longevity and lower incidence of heart disease. My mom has a glass of merlot or cabernet every single night. She truly believes it's her healthiest habit to date. For most of us, alcohol is a part of our culture, and serious problems rarely exist with moderate drinking.

The issue becomes dire when we turn to alcohol to numb our feelings, or we otherwise can't have fun or get through the day without it. Using alcohol as a crutch to cope with life - instead of as a celebratory function - will undoubtedly lead to a host of physical and cognitive problems. Alcohol is essentially a depressant and a dehydrating one at that. You can see the affects of hard drinking on skin, and no amount of makeup or potions can hide this.

Years ago, I attended my ten year high school reunion. Even though all of us were approaching our thirties and still young, the vast range in lifestyles was starkly evident. For the most part, I could deduce which girls partied and binged on vodka sodas on a regular basis just by closely looking at their faces. Their skin looked tired, and I could see fine lines and pores taking shape on pretty, youthful complexions. Of course, sun exposure, age, smoking, and genetics all play a very important role in skin health. None of us are blessed with perfect skin, but heavy alcohol will certainly take its toll by causing excessive dehydration and otherwise negative effects on both the mind and body.

If you happen to suffer from depression, it is best to give up alcohol completely. Depression will never resolve - even with the best treatment - if you habitually worsen your brain chemistry with any amount of alcohol. The brain communicates with a complex system of chemical and electrical signals, which are vital in regulating every aspect of the body's function. These chemical signals are called neurotransmitters and are either excitatory, meaning they stimulate brain activity, or inhibitory, meaning they decrease brain activity. Alcohol increases the effects of the inhibitory neurotransmitter, GABA. Alcohol works as a depressant through this physiological slow-down. The long-term effects of alcohol on the brain can be even more damaging. Most depressed drinkers will feel better even just after one week of abstaining.

Even if you don't suffer from depression, alcohol can cause a whole host of problems including poor sleep, low energy, and weight gain. The liver detoxifies and clears the waste for your body - however, it cannot do its job if it constantly has to process alcohol. Skipping alcohol will not only improve mental clarity, but help keep your body "cleaner" as well.

Most of us are blissfully unaware of just how much alcohol we consume. One drink is equivalent to 12 ounces (1 bottle or can) of beer or wine cooler, 5 ounces (1 glass) of wine, and 1.5 ounces (1 shot) of hard liquor. Pay attention to how much you're consuming by drinking slowly and alternating alcoholic drinks with non-alcoholic drinks at parties.

Nowadays - while I still love an artfully crafted cocktail - I try to choose an organic red wine or a locally made red wine that uses minimal pesticides. Grapes are considered to be one of the "dirtiest" fruit when it comes to pesticides, so wine shouldn't be an exception to a cleaner diet. Red wine - especially pinot noir or wine from cooler regions - is high in resveratrol, an ingredient that touts anti-aging and heart protective benefits. Remember, though, that consuming three or more servings of alcohol is actually associated with worse health, including a modest spike in cancer. Because sometimes it can be hard for me to stop, I'll forgo alcohol on most days. Lastly, "shots" or "shooters" are fun, but really only meant for twenty-one year olds or those on their bachelorette parties. They are a glorified way to get drunk really quickly and can cause unhealthy spikes in blood sugar. Enjoy your drink, but put the kamikazes down!

Day 18
Cook more

If you really don't know how to cook, I urge you to take a couple of lessons at your convenience. Grab a friend or spouse, a bottle of wine, and make a night of it. Or simply just watch some cooking shows on TV or read a recipe book to familiarize yourself with common ingredients and processes. Start with easy meals, and don't give up after failures.

I'm not a gourmet chef, but I've learned to put together a decent meal over the years. I try to remember the basic premise of our home-cooked meals when growing up if I'm having trouble thinking of what to serve - a meat, a vegetable, and a starch. One of my all-time favorite meals is baked salmon with extra virgin olive oil, fresh lemon juice, and seasoning (I try to use wild-caught salmon, since farm raised uses antibiotics). I pair this with bacon-wrapped butternut squash and boil some rice. The meal is so easy to pull off (especially if I cut and wrap the butternut in the morning - that way it is ready to be tossed in the oven by dinner time) but looks elegant enough to serve to guests. Plus, the earthiness of the butternut squash really complements the bacon and salmon.

I've also come to realize that nothing is more emotionally and physically enriching than cooking delicious and nutritious food with my own hands and serving it to loved ones. Additionally, you can shed the excess calories from takeout, save money, and get the opportunity to expose young family members to a variety of tastes and textures. In fact, when people eat more homemade meals, they lower their risk of diabetes by 13 percent and obesity by 15 percent.

Get young children involved in the act of food preparation, as well. They may be more amenable to trying new foods if they participated in the process from start to finish. Take them to farmer's markets and have them pick out their favorite fruits and vegetables. Allow them to do simple tasks like washing or mixing. If they are older, they can cut and use peelers. I always think of a home of being complete when the aroma of something delicious is permeating the air. Kids often remember this too and learn to appreciate home-cooked meals when they get older. In fact, a recipe book of their favorite childhood meals makes the perfect wedding or housewarming gift and will benefit their own family for years to come.

Day 19
Get fresh air, but be mindful of polluted areas

Did you ever notice that children and pets seem to sleep better if they've been outside all day? It is not your imagination. Fresh air is beneficial to your health by cleaning out your lungs and lowering stress levels. Sitting in a windowless office or being cooped up inside all day goes against human nature. We were meant to enjoy the outdoors and appreciate the scenery.

However, we have to pay attention to the air we're breathing and water we're drinking. Major cities are the obvious culprits, but be wary of obscure areas that appear unoffending. Steer clear of locations that house chemical plants, landfills, or storage tanks that emit dangerous toxins into the air or ground. Not only does dirty air cause harm from the inside out, it can actually attack your skin and age you faster than clean air. Sometimes, this can't be avoided. I grew up in heavily refining and industry-laden New Jersey, so I'm aware that we can't escape some pollutants and toxins. But I do urge you to look at city data if you're purchasing a home and are able to choose among a few towns. Even if it means a few extra minutes of commute to work, choose the cleanest possible area to raise your family.

Be wary of your town's water supply, as well. Never rely on tap water unless you know exactly what is in it. Take the element of fluoride, for instance. Fluoride only works to prevent cavities when applied topically to teeth - not ingested - yet towns have been adding this potentially dangerous element to the water supply for years. Stomach upset is the least of our concerns when it comes to too much fluoride. Research has proven that fluoride can affect bone health, thyroid function, and even IQ levels - among a whole host of other health problems. In fact, you would be doing your infant more harm than good if you were to use fluoridated tap water to mix with formula. And never accept a prescription for fluoride-containing vitamins or supplements for your child from your healthcare provider. I used to dispense these all the time years ago and never even batted an eye. We didn't know as much about the dangers of fluoride back then as we do now. If you are interested in learning more about this topic, I urge you to read Dr. Joseph Mercola's article on his website.

Hidden pollution and toxins can also be found in the land that so many homes are built on. My husband and I run into this problem often, because it is our eventual dream to own some semi-rural acreage in which our kids can run around and truly enjoy all that nature has to offer. The problem is that so much of the available land is actually farmland and polluted with the residual toxins and pesticides of harvested crops. Take the great state of Washington, for example. Studies by the Washington Department of Health have shown that children who grow up in the apple-growing region of Central Washington are exposed to more lead than children from any other part of the state. Years ago, these apple orchards were sprayed with lead and arsenate containing pesticides. It was a practice that had a mainstay in apple harvesting for many decades, until it ceased in favor of a safer pesticide. The problem is that lead doesn't break down in soil. Exposure to lead can cause a lot of serious health issues, such as potential cancers, low IQ, and behavioral problems in children. As mentioned before, we can't escape some things. But we can do our part to lower exposure, and soil testing is one way to accomplish this.

Day 20
Protect your heart

Women's heart health is a realm that I'm especially passionate about, only because the numbers are astonishing and truly don't lie. Heart disease is the number one killer of all women, and about 90% of women have one or more risk factors for developing heart disease. Many women fear breast cancer - undeniably an incredible threat - but 1 in 31 women will die from breast cancer, while 1 in 3 women will die from heart disease. That's nearly ten times the risk. We need to start protecting our hearts as soon as possible and learning the factors that contribute to heart disease.

Since heart disease runs rampant on both sides of my family, I know I need to take extra precautions to protect my heart - even though I'm relatively young and ignorance tells me I have years before I should start worrying. My dad first experienced shortness of breath while in his early fifties. Because he caught this in time, his cardiologist was able to perform a double bypass surgery which allowed new arteries to literally "bypass" the diseased sections and increase blood flow to his heart. He remains stable with his medication regimen and regular check-ups with his cardiologist.

The scariest thing about heart disease is that many contributing factors are "silent" and include high blood pressure, high blood sugar, high cholesterol, and even some congenital problems that you may or may not be aware of. Even perfectly healthy women can go about their day with one or more of these issues and not even realize it. Smoking, physical inactivity, and obesity are also major risk factors.

Many of the contributing factors for heart disease are "silent"; even the healthiest of women may not realize they're at risk.

These factors all contribute to a process called *atherosclerosis*, a condition in which plaque builds up in the walls of the arteries and makes it difficult for blood to flow through. Sometimes a blood clot can develop and stop blood flow completely. If this happens, the end result is usually a heart attack or a stroke.

Stress and mental health tend to affect a women's heart

differently than a man's, since these are strongly influenced by hormones and reproductive statuses. In fact, the American Heart Association states that "high blood pressure, migraine with aura, atrial fibrillation, diabetes, depression, and emotional stress are stroke factors that tend to be stronger or more common in woman than in men."

If you're not quite sure where you stand when it comes to cardiovascular health, the Woman's Heart Foundation has an online quiz to help assess your risks. Again, it doesn't matter if you're young, old, healthy, or have a genetic predisposition - every woman has some degree of risk and it's never too early to start paying attention. Here is an adaptation of the quiz:

Do you have a family history of heart disease?
A family history is defined as your father or brother under age 55 or your mother or sister under age 65 having had a heart attack, stroke, angioplasty, or bypass surgery.

Are you of older age?
Older age is defined as over 55 years old. The death rate for cardiovascular diseases increases sharply for women over 65 years old.

Do you smoke?
Or are exposed to second-hand smoke every day?

Do you have high blood pressure?
High blood pressure is defined as 135/85 mm Hg. Or your doctor may have told you that you have high blood pressure in the past. Remember that an optimal blood pressure is 120/80 mm Hg, but many healthcare professionals are now recommending less than that.

Are you physically inactive?
You do not exercise for at least thirty minutes of moderate physical

activity, like taking a brisk walk, on most days.

Do you have diabetes?
You either take medication to control your blood sugar or have been told by a doctor that you have high blood sugar. After age 45, diabetes affects many more women than men.

Do you have high cholesterol?
Elevated lipids are defined as the following parameters:

HDL (your "good" cholesterol) is less than 50mg/dL

LDL-C (your "bad" cholesterol) is over 100mg/dL

Triglycerides are over 150mg/dL

Total cholesterol is over 130mg/dL

*Remember, perfectly healthy women walk around with high cholesterol levels and not even know it. Cholesterol is not just determined by diet, but by genetic predisposition as well.

Are you overweight?
Overweight is defined as 20 pounds greater than your ideal weight.

Do you have metabolic syndrome?
This is an odd term that you may have never heard of before. Metabolic syndrome is defined as having at least three of a cluster of symptoms that are as follows:

High blood sugar greater than 100mg/dL after fasting

High triglycerides (of at least 150mg/dL)

Low HDL levels (less than 50mg/dL)

Blood pressure of 130/85 or greater

Waist circumference over 35 inches

Do you have premature menopause?
Do you have menopause - either natural or surgically induced - that occurred before the age of 40?

*Remember, our hormones play a part in our cardiovascular risk. This is a great risk factor that men generally don't have to worry about.

Are you on the birth control pill?
The birth control greatly increases your risk of heart attack and stroke, especially over the age of 35 and if you concurrently smoke cigarettes. These days, women are now screened for blood pressure issues prior to the prescribing of the birth control pill. I talk more about synthetic hormones in Day 29.

Do you have a high stress level?
Stress is a normal part of our life. Sustained high levels of stress throughout time can damage your heart.

Do you have an unhealthy diet?
The Woman's Heart Foundation defines a healthy diet as this:

Eating fruits, vegetables, and whole-grain, high-fiber foods on a daily basis

Eating fish at least twice a week

Limiting saturated fats (examples are fatty beef, pork, butter, and cheese)

Limiting alcohol to no more than 1 drink per day

Limiting sodium intake (should be less than 1 teaspoonful per day)

Avoiding all *trans* fatty acids (artificial *trans* fat adds hydrogen to liquid vegetable oils to make them more solid and give foods a better taste and texture)

If you answered "yes" to two or more questions, the Woman's Heart Foundation recommends seeing your doctor as soon as possible for a complete risk assessment.

Pre-eclampsia

We can't forget about the blood pressure issues that may arise as a result of pregnancy. Pre-eclampsia - a major blood pressure disorder in pregnancy - doubles the risk of stroke and quadruples the risk of high blood pressure later in life. Many healthcare professionals are now recognizing pre-eclampsia as a major risk factor for cardiovascular disease even well after pregnancy.

If you have high blood pressure before pregnancy, your doctor may consider putting you on aspirin or calcium supplement therapy to lower your risk of developing pre-eclampsia. You may be asking yourself, *Why calcium*? Typically, blood pressure falls during early pregnancy, then slowly rises until the end. However, low calcium intake appears to shift this equilibrium and increase the risk of developing pre-eclampsia. In populations with low calcium intake, the World Health Organization now recommends a daily calcium supplementation to all woman to reduce the risk of pre-eclampsia.

Remember, this calcium supplementation guideline is only for pregnant women and blood pressure. I talk more about calcium supplementation for bone health in Day 23.

Day 21
Realize that most "beautifying" chemicals are toxic

I love wearing cosmetics as much as the next girl. And the times I'm able to sneak off to the nail or hair salon to do something nice for myself are special and often much needed. But the harsh reality is that we need to be more mindful of the chemicals we are willingly placing on our skin, lips, hair, and nails. The fumes emitted and chemicals used in hair and nail salons are toxic no matter how we justify them. Make sure the salon you frequent is well-ventilated. Avoid artificial nails and hair procedures if you're thinking of getting pregnant or are actively pregnant. If you do happen to be pregnant, also try to reduce the amount of spray perfumes and aerosolized hair products used.

Should you work in or own a salon, open the windows as much as possible. Use high quality air filters and replace them often. I know it looks silly to wear a face mask, but do so if you're concerned. You have a right to be. When it comes to permanent hair dye, the FDA in the United States still permits carcinogens and other toxic synthetic chemicals, while Europe has banned them. These chemicals include aminophenol, diaminobenzene, and phenyledediamine. One study has found that hairdressers - who are exposed to more hair dye than the rest of us - have a 27 percent higher risk of lung cancer, 30 percent greater risk of bladder cancer, and 62 percent increased risk of multiple myeloma. These are substantial numbers and serious risks!

As far as cosmetics, I know how hard it is to switch out the items that we're accustomed to and feel that work for us. It may have taken since our awkward teenage years to find the suitable brands and palettes! If nothing else, at least consider switching to a healthier lipstick. Accurate scientific data is lacking, but it is estimated that women swallow an exorbitant amount of lipstick throughout their lifetime. Whether the purported statistics are exaggerated or not, lipstick is undoubtedly easily ingested and potentially enters the bloodstream. Look for alternate brands that contain organic, plant-based ingredients and very few petrochemicals, parabens, sulfates, and pthalates. One of my favorite cosmetic brands is Tarte, which uses naturally-derived ingredients.

You don't have to go crazy and do a complete overhaul on your vanity. Just realize that anything we put on our skin has the potential to be absorbed into our body. This same notion applies even more so to babies and young children whose skin is thinner and much more delicate than ours. If you're not quite sure where to begin, your local health food store is a great resource for more natural alternatives.

Day 22
Stop habitually being late

Traffic happens. Kids puke on their clothes. Hair dryers mysteriously stop working. Life happens, and we have all been on late on occasion. But if you are habitually late to meetings, dinner dates, doctor's appointments, and - Heaven forbid - even work or school, you have to start realizing the amount of disrespect you are unintentionally and unfortunately showing to people. Plus - disrespect aside - I personally develop an inherent stress whenever I am running behind. I feel as though I need to rush, which leads to the almost inevitable fact that I'll forget something, experience some sort of wardrobe malfunction, or make a wrong turn. I get so flustered that I'm certain people can sense my jumpiness when I finally do arrive. Giving myself extra time allows me to relax, get my proverbial ducks in a row, and put on my best face possible before venturing out into the world. Especially when it comes to stressful events, having the time to take a few deep breaths is everything to me.

Several researchers and scientists have conducted studies on habitually late people to determine their attributes and reasons for their lackadaisical attitude towards schedules. Many of these studies have revealed that people who are late tend to be more creative, optimistic, and even experience better longevity. One study even found an actual time misperception between Type A and Type B personalities. For Type A personalities - the more high-strung of the two subtypes - a minute passed by in 58 seconds, whereas Type B personalities felt a minute pass in 77 seconds. The conductor of the study stated that these extra 18 seconds can add up over time. So there really is a science behind lateness!

While late people may have some positive traits that help explain their tendency, it is estimated that lateness costs the American economy millions of dollar per year in lost productivity. Time is the most precious commodity we have. If time becomes valorized, everyone wins.

If you have to dupe yourself in believing that events start twenty minutes earlier than they really do, start doing so. Other helpful tips include packing bags or lunches, showering, and laying out clothes the night before. Pay attention to traffic and weather reports and prepare accordingly. Give every effort to be on time. Arriving when expected not only shows that you're honorable enough to keep your word, but also considerate enough to think of other people. You never know what strings the other party had to pull to be there, too.

Day 23
Take vitamin D

If you are to only take one supplement in life, make it vitamin D. The vast majority of us are deficient in this all-encompassing, multi-beneficial nutrient - so much so, that the lack of it may be contributing to certain health issues and diseases. Vitamin D has many health advantages including promoting bone health; normalizing blood pressure; facilitating the immune system; warding off depression; and reducing risks of certain cancers, heart disease, and diabetes. For women especially, adequate intake of vitamin D is essential for preventing osteoporosis. Many drugs for osteoporosis - while still regarded as safe amongst the medical community - have a whole host of side effects and potential dangers that make it difficult for many women to take. These drugs also make thick, but weak bones. We need to start paying attention to our bones way beforehand, and this includes supplementing with vitamin D.

The void of vitamin D in most lifestyles is very difficult to make up with dietary choices and sun exposure. Almost all of us require a supplement to get the recommended daily amount. Many of us who live further north - 40 degrees north latitude, to be more specific - probably won't make any vitamin D in the winter due to decreases in sunlight exposure. So for about 5 months of the year, northern inhabitants are deficient in one of the most important nutrients possible for our bodies! In fact, seasonal affective disorder or low mood during the winter months have long been linked to deficiencies in vitamin D. This theory makes complete sense when you consider the amount of vitamin D receptors found in brain and nerve tissue.

Many discrepancies exist regarding the right dosage of vitamin D to take. Too much vitamin D can harm your kidneys and be toxic. I generally recommend 1000 to 2000 IUs of vitamin D3 daily, which is better absorbed by the body than vitamin D2. This dose seems to be a fair balance among the literature available.

Calcium - A Dichotomy

When many of us hear the words *bone health*, an almost Pavlov-like reaction is to secondarily think *calcium*. From the time we were little children, we've been told that drinking our milk would help make us stronger in order to outrun little Jimmy in dodge-ball, jump higher in cheer tryouts, or do whatever other physical feat we set out to accomplish. Undeniably, this notion still holds true. Eating foods rich in calcium will help keep our bones strong and healthy.

The discrepancy lies in calcium supplements, as a growing

number of healthcare professionals are not routinely recommending them as a way to prevent osteoporosis. Here's why: when it comes to calcium (and some other *nutraceuticals*), our bodies can only absorb so much. In fact, the more calcium we consume, the less our bodies will absorb, and most of this calcium will be excreted in our urine.

Hormones such as growth hormone, estrogen, testosterone, and parathyroid hormone control how much calcium is deposited in our bones. This is why calcium supplementation alone is not a great way to "fool" our body into absorbing more calcium - our hormones are actually in charge of this. An excellent way to stimulate these hormones is through weight-bearing exercises. Vitamin D can also help increase the amount of calcium our bodies absorb.

Here is the dichotomy with calcium: calcium supplementation in men has been linked to prostate cancer, however can lower the risk of developing colon cancer. Calcium has also been shown to both worsen and improve cardiovascular disease. Why the dichotomy? Pharmacist, Gunda Siska, explains it perfectly in an article she wrote for the *Pharmacy Times*.

" I have seen this dichotomy of results several times. It is a pattern that occurs with some, but not all, nutraceuticals. It is my belief that this is occurring because when a nutritional deficiency is restored to normal, miraculous health benefits occur; conversely, when normal levels are elevated even higher with synthetic supplements, good things rarely happen and sometimes bad things happen.

It is my belief that the study outcome results are dependent on the nutritional status of the participants at the start of the study. If the participant is poorly nourished, they will benefit from the nutraceutical. If they are well nourished, and they take synthetic nutraceutical pills then they do not benefit, and they may have a bad outcome such as cancer or accelerated cardiovascular disease."

So what do we do when it comes to preventing osteoporosis? I like recommending a natural method of weight-bearing exercises, a diet rich in calcium, and taking vitamin D to help increase the amount of calcium ingested through the diet. Recreational activities like smoking and drinking alcohol also play a huge role in decreasing bone mass density and should try to be limited as much as possible. In fact, smoking has been shown to decrease bone mass density at all skeletal sites.

If you suspect you may have weak bones, a bone density test is recommended. You can also check your serum levels of vitamin D, as well.

A Word on Osteoporosis Medications

Our bones constantly go through a renewal cycle where breakdown and restoration occur almost at the same rate. Osteoporosis happens when breakdown occurs more than restoration, resulting in a reduction of bone mass and bone tissue deterioration. Bisphosphonates - drugs like Fosamax and Boniva - are presently considered first-line medication therapy for osteoporosis and work by stopping bone breakdown. But bisphosphonates have some very real risks, and about half of all patients taking them will eventually stop due to the side effects. Side effects include back and joint pain, nausea, vomiting, constipation, and heartburn. Bisphosphonates also create a denser bone, which in theory sounds optimal for treating osteoporosis. But this denser bone doesn't remodel well and allow for good blood supply. So we see more serious, albeit rare, side effects like jaw necrosis - bone tissue death that can't be treated - and femoral fractures. By interfering with the natural cycle of bone breakdown, these drugs may sometimes do more harm than good.

Bisphosphonates do have a place in treatment for osteoporosis - especially in elderly women whose osteoporosis has been well established - but this is a condition in which prevention really is key. Because osteoporosis tends be age-related, take advantage of the time you have to protect and save your bones. Decreasing caffeine intake to less than 3 cups of coffee per day, partaking in exercise with strength and balance training, and getting adequate exposure to sunlight all help to prevent osteoporosis.

Day 24
Stand up straight

Proper posture can make you look 10 pounds lighter, appear more confident, and align your body in such a way as to avoid strain to the supporting muscles and ligaments. I constantly have to remind myself to stand up straight. Between my line of work, lugging small children around, and bending over to change diapers and clothes, it is very tempting for me to be in continual slouch mode. My back definitely feels the physical pain of improper posture. I even look tired and defeated when I'm hunched. Sure, I may *feel* tired and defeated at any given time, but at least I don't have to look it!

If you sit at a desk all day, pay attention to how you sit and make it a point to get up and walk around when you can. When sitting, make sure your feet are flat on the ground, legs uncrossed, and your head is stretched towards the ceiling. Consciously thinking about how we sit or stand can help prevent a lot of unnecessary back issues and have profound cosmetic benefits.

Day 25
Eat as colorfully and organically as possible, and try to avoid genetically modified ingredients (GMOs)

I'm not a nutritionist and have never subscribed to any sort of diet - but my love for food is practically tangible, and I've learned how to have a good relationship with it in order to live a productive and functioning life. Look at food for the nutrients it offers - not the fat and calories - and you will inherently make better choices.

"Medicine is not healthcare. Food is healthcare. Medicine is sick care."

Diseases and illnesses find it difficult to thrive in healthy, well-nourished body. Proper nutrition is undeniably proper healthcare.

"Eat the rainbow" and try to incorporate colors at least five times a day. Look for options that make this easier to achieve - like fruit smoothies, big salads, or roasted vegetables with olive oil and your favorite seasonings. If you can fill your plate with more healthy stuff, it will leave less room for junk. I eat well and like a variety of temptations, so I won't lie and say it's easy to maintain a trim waistline. In fact, my waistline is probably anything but trim. But I feel strong and healthy and like the way my clothes fit most of the time, so I count these achievements as positives.

The United States has much more lenient requirements for pesticide levels than other countries, so we need to be especially mindful of the potentially toxic chemicals that we are unnecessarily ingesting. Try to eat as organically as possible, and don't just stop at fruits and vegetables. Meat and dairy products should also have limited amounts of hormones, antibiotics, and pesticides. I know that procuring such items can be expensive. Even just switching out a couple of items that you eat regularly will help. Buy meats in bulk if you can and freeze. Frozen organic fruits and vegetables are great options, too. And shop local if you have the option to. Local farmers tend to use less pesticides and chemicals, since the time and travel associated from harvesting to selling is minimal.

The "Dirty Dozen" and "Clean Fifteen"

Each year, the Environmental Working Group (EWG) analyzes data from the U.S Department of Agriculture and the Food and Drug Administration to determine the pesticide levels for common fruits and vegetables. Some produce is exposed to more contaminants than others. The "Dirty Dozen" list contains the fruits and vegetables that have the highest loads of pesticide residues. These items should be bought organically whenever possible.

The "Dirty Dozen"

1. Strawberries

2. Spinach

3. Nectarines

4. Apples

5. Peaches

6. Pears

7. Cherries

8. Grapes

9. Celery

10. Tomatoes

11. Sweet bell peppers

12. Potatoes

The "Clean Fifteen"

These fruits and vegetables have been found to contain the least amount of pesticide residues. If buying organic is difficult, you can feel safe that these products are "clean."

1. Sweet corn (However, a lot of corn is genetically modified - read below. Buying organic is your safest bet.)

2. Avocadoes

3. Pineapples

4. Cabbage

5. Onions

6. Frozen sweet peas

7. Papaya

8. Asparagus

9. Mangoes

10. Eggplant

11. Honeydew melon

12. Kiwi

13. Cantaloupe

14. Cauliflower

15. Grapefruit

It's okay if you don't always have these lists handy. Try and pick out a few fruits and vegetables that you or your family consume a lot of and keep those in mind the next time you grocery shop. From the "dirty dozen" list, the largest culprits for our family are spinach, grapes, strawberries, and potatoes - so I always try to remember to buy organic when it comes to those items. Thinking outside of the box is also helpful. For instance, my older son could make a meal out of ketchup alone. For some reason, he just really, really likes ketchup. Since tomatoes carry a lot of pesticides, I've started buying organic ketchup - that is, until he moves on to the next condiment. He also drinks a lot of apple juice. Therefore, I try to buy organic apple juice made with apples grown in the U.S. whenever possible.

I tend to think that any produce with a thick skin will have trouble absorbing substantial amounts of pesticides, so that is also another helpful tip for me when shopping. I almost never feel the need to buy organic when it comes to avocadoes or bananas, two other produce items that we consume a lot of. In fact, many of the products in my pantry are probably not organic. And on those nights that I'm too tired or busy to cook, we do our fair share of takeout and eating at restaurants. I can't be strict with everything all of the time. As long as I pay attention to the biggest culprits for my family, I'm doing my part to lower exposure to harmful chemicals. And if I can't buy organic produce, I'm always careful to wash very thoroughly.

Speaking of children, here is an example of what mine eat in day. I decided to include a child's menu because their diet is actually not that drastically different from mine (for now, at least, and hopefully into adulthood). However, I know how particular children can be and how difficult - and sometimes expensive - this can make grocery shopping, especially if trying to buy good foods on a budget. Many times I'm left scratching my head figuring out what to serve that satisfies everyone's taste buds. Much of the time, I go through the effort of preparing food that's not even eaten. The best thing I can do is lead by example and hope they follow suit.

You will see that I'm not very strict, however I do try to steer clear of foods that are specifically marketed for kids, as these tend to be filled with sugar and preservatives. These foods are also highly tempting to the adults in the household.

Sample Toddler/Child Menu

Breakfast:

Stonyfield Farms yogurt smoothie
sliced banana
half of a cinnamon raisin bagel with cream cheese

OR

scrambled eggs
a few slices of brie or mozzarella cheese
grapes or blueberries

OR

peanut butter toast
apple slices

Lunch:

Egg salad with hard-boiled eggs and little bit of mayonnaise
half an English muffin
slices of cucumber and tomato

OR

Applegate uncured hot dog
handful of kettle-cooked or baked chips
boiled carrots

Dinner:

chicken meatloaf
baked sweet potato "fries"

OR

turkey meatballs with pasta, ricotta cheese, and red sauce

OR

shredded chicken on a tortilla with salsa, sour cream, and cheese
avocado slices

Dessert:

frozen yogurt or fruit bar

OR

chocolate pudding with peaches, strawberries and whipped cream

Snacks:

any kind of fresh fruit or vegetable, yogurt, cheese, peanut-butter
crackers, or pretzels

I hardly ever say "no" to the occasional chips, cookies, or other junk food, except if its right before dinnertime. My rule of thumb is if I choose to purchase and keep those items in the house, then my children have every right to call "dibs" on them. I just try to not let them go crazy.

My son goes through phases of eating everything in sight to not touching anything at all. He is a toddler, so his taste buds are still developing, and he doesn't quite know what satisfies him yet. My job is to present him with quality food, offer him choices, and allow for some autonomy in the whole process - not force-feed him the most nutritious foods in a meager attempt to keep him healthy. I try to stay pretty flexible, and if I can't be perfect, neither can he.

Returning to adults, we have to be extra careful with corn and soy products, as well. While I love a good Mexican restaurant, up to 90 percent of corn - the base ingredient for most chips and tortillas - is genetically modified! The act of creating a GMO is an artificial process in which the genes from the DNA of one plant or species is extracted and forcibly introduced into the DNA of another. In the agricultural industry, genetically modifying corn has allowed for crops that are resistant to pests, disease, or drought. The process can also increase the yield harvested, which means more can be sold. Very drastic views of GMOs exist, including scientists who advocate the process and claim it's harmlessness and anti-GMO activists who are wholeheartedly against them. We just don't have enough data to see the effects of long term GMO consumption to advocate the use, especially in children whose bodies are actively growing and changing. In fact, many other developed countries have stricter limits or even full-fledged bans on foods with GMOs.

Another option that I like is using frozen organic fruits and vegetables. You may be wondering if frozen is as healthy as fresh. Generally speaking, frozen is sometimes even better than fresh, since it is harvested at the peak of freshness and then flash frozen to preserve the integrity and nutrient content of the food. Conversely, fresh food may spend a lot of time in the transit process, thereby losing nutrients from the time it was harvested.

Food will always be a source of comfort to me - and almost everyone else, for that matter - despite my best efforts to deny this. The notion explains why I can't seem to stomach a raw salad during those stark, cold winter months - yet crave fresh, juicy watermelon on a sweltering day in August. It is why the taste of Andes mint chocolates always brings me back to my grandmother's house in Northeast Philly, where she would keep them in beautiful glass dishes around the holidays. Taste is a major sensory perception that goes hand in hand with our sense of smell. Our highly sensitive taste buds actually undergo a chemical reaction that travels to the back of the brain whenever they come in contact with food molecules. No wonder good food has the ability to stimulate other feelings and fond memories.

So what do I do when January comes around in the Northeast, and the sight of raw vegetables and salads actually repels me? I rely heavily on soups, stews, and vegetable-filled casseroles. This is the time of year when my slow-cooker becomes a permanent fixture on my countertop. One of the easiest meals for me to prepare in the morning is a hearty soup in which I dump a bunch of vegetables, bone broth, pulled rotisserie chicken or some other meat, and seasonings into the slow-cooker and let it simmer all day. Pair it with toasted French bread, and the meal is suitable for all family members. I also like creamy vegetable soups, such as butternut squash soup or cream of asparagus. Making these types of soups requires the use of an immersion blender, but that quite literally is the most difficult step.

Creamy Butternut Squash Soup

Butternut squash is known as the "apple of God" - and for good reason. This super-food is loaded with fiber, potassium, magnesium, and beta-carotene - a compound that has antioxidant activity and can help protect cells from damage. I also consumed this soup during the last trimester of my pregnancies, per the advice of my midwife to increase my beta carotene intake. Some evidence exists that beta carotene is helpful in strengthening the amniotic sac, in order to prevent water breaking prematurely - and thus early labor.

My family has come to relate the smell of this soup to chilly fall days, when this hearty, golden concoction is the perfect remedy for

---

my kid's chilly noses and red cheeks from running in the leaves all day. Substitute the cream cheese with coconut milk if you prefer vegan or a lower calorie recipe.

Ingredients

1 package of frozen chopped butternut squash, thawed (can use fresh butternut squash, either 1/2 of a small squash or 16 ounces)

1-2 cups baby carrots

1 small white onion, chopped

2 cups vegetable stock

Fresh, grated ginger to taste (or ginger powder)

Fresh, grated garlic to taste (or garlic powder)

Pinch of nutmeg

Salt and pepper to taste

1 package of low-fat cream cheese (or substitute with about 3/4 cups coconut milk if vegan recipe preferred)

Directions

Place squash, carrots, onion, and seasoning in slow cooker and cook on high for about 4 hours or low for 8 hours. Vegetables should be soft and easily cut. Once the vegetables are cooked, add either cream cheese or coconut milk to make the soup creamy. Chop the cream cheese into smaller pieces and place in crock pot (or add the coconut milk if preferred). Using an immersion blender, or transferring batches to a regular blender, blend everything until smooth and creamy. Additional broth may added to adjust the consistency to your liking. Garnish with pumpkin seeds or coconut milk.

Everything in moderation

When it comes to keeping an overall healthy, well-balanced diet, try an 80/20 or a 5-day/2-day rule. This simply means eating well during the weekdays and easing up a little on the weekends. Some women I know go as far as to avoid all breads and pastas during the workweek, but I'm usually not that strict. Eating this way allows for zero guilt or regret for weekend indulgences. You never feel deprived and can live your life by going to your favorite restaurants and eating your favorite foods - just not every day of the week. If you follow a somewhat modified rule, never let one indulgence ruin the rest of your day. If you go heavy one meal, go light the next. I like this rule, because it embodies balance and is the most realistic way to live without deprivation.

My Take on "Performance-Enhancing" Products and Supplements

Much abuzz surrounds protein shakes, "detox" pills and teas, and other items marketed as fitness or performance-enhancing supplements these days. These products are sold everywhere from the local pharmacy to health stores and even private sellers or health coaches who believe the product has helped them to achieve their fitness goals and feel it may help you too. I'm not insinuating that these products are necessarily harmful; I actually consume a high-quality protein shake from time to time in order to support muscle and skin health. However, the healthiest, easiest, and most inexpensive way for our bodies to absorb nutrients is through the consumption of whole, unprocessed foods. Many of these products contain chemicals made up in the lab, such as sugar substitutes, coloring, and artificial flavoring.

Some products do have scientific backing. Research exists that support the use of branch-chain amino acids (BCAAs). When taken as an oral supplement during a high-intensity workout, BCAAs can help with cellular growth, proliferation, and repair. The best BCAAs on the market contain leucine, isoleucine, and valine.

I do, however, want you to ask some important questions before forking over the money and expecting to see instantaneous results from expensive products that claim to boost energy, take the bloat out of your tummy, or otherwise be a "panacea" for your nutrition goals - without doing much else.

Since these products are not overseen by the FDA, what are the quality assurance steps that are taken by the manufacturer to ensure that each product has 100% safe ingredients and in the right amounts at all times?

Is there accurate clinical data available to show that these products are superior to placebo in burning calories, giving energy, or whatever else their claim may be?

What does each ingredient do and where does it come from?

For a "detox" product, the liver and kidney already do the best job of ridding toxins from our body (so long as we've retained proper organ function.) How is this product facilitating what our bodies are naturally meant to do?

Think about the cost of the product and how much you feel it is really worth. Do you believe the markup on the product is too high? Remember that the sellers need a profit too, but how much is too much?

You might never know the answer to the last question, but it's worth contemplating as to not waste too much of your money.

To stress the importance of how unregulated these products are, a recent case comes to mind in which the FDA discovered that some companies have been illegally selling mis-labled body building supplements that actually contain steroids or steroid-like substances. The FDA only discovered this finding after people suffered adverse effects from these steroid-containing products over the course of seven years. Some adverse effects were very serious including liver and kidney injuries, heart attack, stroke, and male infertility. Many cases required hospitalization. Again, the FDA is not required to monitor these products, however they will eventually step in if adverse events are being noted - but, often times, it is too late and many people have already been affected. Undeniably, this was a serious case and doesn't represent the vast majority of reputable products that do abide by good manufacturing processes.

Again - rarities aside - I don't think these products are necessarily harmful and actually believe that some protein powders and other supplements are beneficial in the realm of competitive training or professional sports. As a healthcare professional, I can't champion these products; however, I also don't discourage their use if you feel they are working for you and helping you to be in good physical shape. But, as with everything else in life, you have the right to ask some questions and not waste your money. Remember, some companies use low-quality ingredients that our bodies have trouble absorbing, simply because the FDA is not monitoring them. "Energy" products can also mask the root cause of lethargy and fatigue. A cup of coffee contains similar amounts of caffeine found in many energy products and is cheaper and easier.

Moderation is key with these products. Not many things - including a multi-million dollar industry - can take the place of a nutritious, well-balanced diet. For the average consumer whose sole purpose is to look and feel a little better, you may find that not much benefit is derived from expensive products that are "celebrity-endorsed" or have an eye-catching package design.

Day 26
Take tips from women of other cultures

I attended college in an urban setting and was subsequently exposed to a lot of different cultures during those years. After college, I went on to work for a large company which expanded my experiences with diversity even more. I found it interesting that these hard working women from different parts of the world always seemed like they had it more "together" than my fellow American peers who frequently seemed to be stressed out or chasing pipe dreams. Looking back, I know that wasn't really the case. We all had it "together" in our own special way. But perhaps it was just intriguing to observe the different way these women approached life and their unique views on the world. They had an air of mystique which prompted me to look with admiring eyes. I wanted to listen to their stories and learn about how they lived in an effort to better my own life.

In many ways, women all around the world share an unique thread that unifies and connects us to each other. But truth to be told, learning and embracing the differences in other cultures can teach us a lot about life, careers, motherhood, and just about everything in between. Culturally diverse women may not always be "right" in their ways, but we can take a lot of positive aspects from everyone's heritage and intertwine them with our own philosophies and beliefs to live a more a cultured and sophisticated life. I love reading self-help books from worldly authors or from women who spent time in a different country and really learned their culture. We become enlightened when we open our minds and see things in a different light or try new ways of doing things. Most adaptations can be fairly simple.

For instance, you may try and incorporate more exotic spices in your cooking like the Indian women do. Turmeric has long been used for a myriad of health benefits due to the active component, *curcumen*. This powerful spice can fight inflammation, act as an antioxidant, protect the heart, and potentially fight against diabetes and cancers. Other commonly used spices in Indian cooking include cardamom, saffron, coriander, and clove - all of which can be attributable to optimum health.

Golden Tea Recipe

There's nothing more comforting to the soul than a hot cup of tea. I am a big tea drinker and have found that some herbal preparations are even more soothing than a glass of wine at night. Among my favorites are matcha green tea (loaded with antioxidants), chamomile (known for its calming properties), and chai (an Indian favorite). The following recipe for "golden tea" tastes very similar to chai and contains turmeric, which gives it a beautiful golden color. All of the other ingredients have numerous health benefits as well. If you suffer from any sort of inflammation, try drinking this creamy and delicious remedy as a midday or evening treat.

2 cups coconut milk

A pinch of ground cinnamon

1/2 teaspoon dried turmeric

Thinly sliced fresh ginger (enough for your liking)

1 tablespoon raw, unfiltered honey

1/4 teaspoon whole, black peppercorns (this is optional - black peppercorn is purported to enhance the absorption of turmeric)

Mix all ingredients in a saucepan and simmer for about 10 minutes. Simmering will help meld the flavors together. Pour through a strainer and enjoy. You can also make extra and store in the refrigerator in an airtight container for up to 5 days. Reheat before serving.

You could even take a few style tips from French women in order to look effortlessly *chic*. In "The French Beauty Solution," author Mathilde Thomas recommends a "done-but-not-done" look. Start with well-maintained, hydrated skin and use makeup to play up one feature at a time. French women rarely use eyeshadow, but believe in well-groomed eyebrows. Lips are softly dressed up with classic colors, like dusty rose or classic red. Hair is kept natural and not over-processed with colors and heat. This simplistic approach to beauty focuses on foundational maintenance and accepting and even playing-up your flaws.

In fact, let's start taking tips from *all* women - no matter their background - whom we admire and believe are happy and confident. Suppose you know a woman at work who is always fashionable and well-groomed. Aesthetics aside, she appears to excel at everything she touches both professionally and non. She's smart, confident, and capable. Instead of truly appreciating her qualities, how many of you would have negative, self-deprecating thoughts? I'll stop and run through a list of some of them, because even I am no stranger to self-doubts and succumb to these notions at times. *She only looks that way because she can afford fancy clothes and beauty treatments. She knows the boss - that's the only reason she got the job. Sure, she does good work, but only because she doesn't have any kids at home that drain her time and energy. Maybe if I had the money for a top-notch education, I could be in her position too.*

Do these types of thoughts sound familiar? *They stem from self-doubt.* If I ever find myself making excuses and jumping to conclusions, I first tell myself to try and look past the obvious. For instance, I'll refer to the above notion that lack of kids give this woman an edge at work. What if she's been struggling with infertility for years, but she puts on a strong face professionally to hide her personal hardship? What if she cries with every failed pregnancy test? What if she sees a tired, overworked mother with her three kids at the supermarket and would give anything to experience that?

I know I'm not the first person to make a wrong assumption in my quest to cover my own self-doubts. Instead of taking the negative path, we need to start appreciating the good qualities from other women and see how we can apply those strengths to our own lives. Instead of getting caught up in self-deprecation, let's emerge ourselves in self-motivation. If we see a strong, successful woman, ask yourself *what can she teach me?* I guarantee that positive things will happen the minute we transform our thoughts and start appreciating and learning from the great qualities of others.

Day 27
Take a probiotic

Our digestive tract is truly amazing. The vast majority of our entire immune system is located in our digestive tract, as well as a good deal of our neurological system. In fact, there are more serotonin receptors in our gut than in our actual brain! It makes sense that having a healthy gut can exhibit an overall beneficial effect on our wellbeing. Adding a probiotic can help restore and optimize digestive health by increasing the ratio of good to bad bacteria. And a daily probiotic is absolutely necessary if you are on chronic proton pump inhibitor (PPI) therapy for acid reflux, prolonged antibiotic therapy, or any kind of regimen that suppresses the immune system.

The immunity benefits offered by probiotics are astounding. The microbial community found in our guts is referred to as the *microbiome*, which plays a vital role in our immune response. If the balance of good and bad bacteria is off, we are at risk for developing diseases that affect our whole body - not just the gastrointestinal tract. Supporting the microbiome through the use of probiotics is a healthy, alternative way to keep illnesses at bay.

Probiotics support the microbiome through several mechanisms. First, they act as a physical barrier, lining the intestinal tract and fighting against harmful bacteria. They also support the intestinal tract's mucus layer, enhancing mucus production which serves as protection. Lastly, probiotics support and strengthen the cells that help remove foreign substances.

Probiotics are also helpful if you suffer from any sort of gastrointestinal disorder, such as irritable bowel syndrome or "leaky gut" syndrome - an unconventional diagnosis in which damage to the intestinal lining causes bacteria and other toxins to "leak out" into the bloodstream. "Leaky gut" syndrome can lead to host of problems including abdominal bloating, painful gas/cramps, food sensitivities, joint paint, rashes, and autoimmune disorders. By taking a probiotic, you can reduce intestinal inflammation, normalize gut dysfunction, and alleviate hypersensitivity reactions.

While it may seem that probiotics are a new fangled idea these days, the notion couldn't be further from the truth. Many of our ancestors thrived on probiotics found in fermented and cultured foods long before the invention of refrigerators. In fact, because of refrigeration, it is pretty difficult to find probiotics in food these days and most likely has to be supplemented in the typical American diet.

Increasing the amount of probiotics in your diet can be accomplished by consuming yogurt, kefir, miso, or even sauerkraut. Also, adding a couple tablespoonfuls of apple cider vinegar on a regular basis can create an acid level that supports the growth of probiotics.

If you're not amenable to the above dietary additions, look for a reputable supplement. Probiotics are measured in CFUs and, in general, the higher the CFU count, the more effective it will be. Probiotics with at least 15 billion CFUs are recommended. Also, look for a decent amount of diverse strains, of which 1 or 2 of those strains should be the kind that ensure the probiotic gets to the gut and is able to colonize without being destroyed by stomach acid. Protective strains such as these include *bacillus coagulans, saccharomyces boulardii, bacillus subtilis,* and *lactobacillus rhamnosus.*

Other Ways to Improve the Microbiome

Take 2 tablespoonfuls of raw apple cider vinegar per day

Raw apple cider vinegar (ACV) has many health benefits due to its powerful healing compounds which include acetic acid, potassium, magnesium, and enzymes. Studies have shown that ACV can promote weight loss by reducing sugar cravings and promoting detoxification. Try taking two tablespoonfuls before eating a large meal or going out to eat. The acetic acid in ACV is also natural antibiotic, in that it has the ability to kill "bad bacteria" while promoting "good bacteria" growth. Because of this property, ACV can be used for fungal infections, colds, and sore throats. The acetic acid can also lower body pH, which can be helpful for reducing chronic illnesses like cancer, high blood pressure, and diabetes.

I always keep a bottle of ACV on hand and take two tablespoonfuls of it a day. The kind I buy also contains a bunch of organic herbs and spices such as ginseng, Echinacea, ginger, and fenugreek. I'll be honest - the initial few gulps are a little hard to get down. Now that I am accustomed to the taste and know what to expect, the bitterness has actually grown on me in a weird way! When buying ACV, make sure it is raw, organic, unfiltered, and with the "mother" intact, which means it contains all of the original beneficial compounds. ACV may appear cloudy or murky with web-like components, but this is actually a good thing. The strands are actually bits of live yeast that contain helpful bacteria, and the cloudiness simply means that all the enzymes and active components are still intact.

ACV has many other uses and includes the following:

Makes hair shine (mix a tablespoonful in a cup of water and apply after shampooing, then wash out)

Naturally whitens teeth (rub on teeth and let stand for a minute)

Tones the skin and helps with eczema and acne (apply topically to skin, then wash off)

Helps with toenail fungus (apply to fungus twice a day)

Works as a natural deodorant (dab on armpits)

Decrease sugar and artificial sweeteners

Decreasing the amount of both sugar and artificial sweeteners from your diet can also improve the microbiome. Sugars are easily absorbed from the intestines, without any help of your good microbes. Sugar tends to feed the bad bacteria, as opposed to the good bacteria.

Increase your intake of fruits and vegetables

A diet rich in diverse fruits and vegetables will help create a microbiome diverse in good bacteria. Focus on green leafy vegetables, asparagus, and carrots. Foods like garlic and turmeric are also helpful.

Decrease your alcohol and caffeine intake

I may be starting to sound like a broken record, but consuming large amounts of "uppers" and "downers" will be a big downfall to your overall health - not just gut health. Alcohol and caffeine are notorious for being harsh on the stomach and will worsen any ulcer or underlying inflammation.

Day 28
Get moving

A day in the life of many Americans means sitting at a job for 8 hours a day, sitting in an hour of traffic coming home, sitting at the dinner table to eat, then maybe sitting on the couch to watch TV for an hour or so before bed. That's a lot of sitting. This was my life not too long ago too, only it was 10 hours a day sitting in a windowless cubicle. If I didn't get a chance to walk around during my lunch break, I was downright miserable. I knew my body wasn't made for that life. No one's body is, yet so many of us fail to get up and get moving. Humans are designed to be functional, even if that means just being able to run in an airport to catch a plane or carry bags of groceries up the flights of stairs in apartment buildings. Our muscles were meant to be used, or else we will lose them. For women especially, muscle tone naturally decreases with age as our metabolism slows down and our cells grow tired. In fact, we lose about five pounds of muscle every decade. We need to fight this process by staying active and toning our muscles.

I'll be the first to admit that I'm no athlete. I dabbled in softball growing up and was always adequate enough for physical fitness testing in gym class, but that's pretty much the extent of my athleticism. I put exercise in the same category as other mandatory chores, like going to the dentist or emptying the dishwasher. I know I have to do it, but I don't exactly derive pleasure from it. My apathy towards exercise may explain while I'll never be a hard body. I much rather tone my body doing something fun, like going for a bike ride or dancing. My sister, Christina, is the exact polar opposite. She owns a fitness studio in California and took first place in a fitness competition, where she sported nothing but a sparkling bikini and high heels on stage in front of thousands of people. She was also over 35 years old at the time and had two children, mind you. She is a great example of completely transforming your body and is the epitome of peak physical health.

While my admiration for my sister never ceases to desist, I have absolutely zero aspirations to wear a bikini on stage. But I do want to be strong and energetic enough for my kids. I want good muscle tone, because I know muscle burns calories even at rest. But most importantly, I want to give the aging process a good fight. My muscles need to know that I still need them and appreciate them even through menopause and beyond.

If you enjoy the workout and find inspiration from group activities, try regularly attending a class or fitness group. Remember the sense of community I discussed on Day 4? Other women can be your greatest motivator, and classes may give you a chance to step outside your regular world, socialize, and have some fun. I will admit that I had the best time years ago at one of my sister's bootcamps. Since I was visiting California from New Jersey, I was the odd man out when everyone paired up for partner exercises. I instantly grabbed my 7 year old niece who was puttering around the gym and asked her to be my partner. We giggled at each other the whole time and had a blast. I can't always work out with my little niece (she's 3,000 miles away, plus I'm sure she would much rather be doing other things), so I have to find other ways to make exercise more enjoyable. I often remind myself that I just have to *move* somehow, someway, every single day. I like to put my headphones on and just go for a walk. Walking is actually one of the most effective ways to tone your legs and rear and is also easy on the joints, making it an excellent workout for those with injury or those in their golden years. I really do try and aim for 10,000 steps a day. A smartwatch or pedometer is a great way to measure how much you actually move. Parking far away and taking the stairs whenever possible are great ways to add to your steps.

Since I have small children at home, I have to find creative ways to incorporate strength training. I've lost some of my core strength due to a couple of pregnancies within a short period of time, so I try and focus on that area along with other problematic zones for me. I sneak in repetitions of planks, lunges, and squats whenever my children are napping or - heaven forbid - actually playing nicely together. Sometimes I try and wake up early and sneak in a quick 20 minute workout from YouTube videos or from the TV. My favorite fitness videos from YouTube are from PopSugar fitness and can usually be completed from start to finish within a half hour. I do these right in the family room and with just a pair of hand weights, and let me tell you, I am usually left sweating profusely and out of breath.

I enrolled one of my sons in a mommy-and-me class at our local Little Gym. The purpose of the class is to provide a social atmosphere and enforce some basic motor skills for the developing toddler. I like to go so my son can safely release some of his energy in a highly padded environment with minimal escape routes.

While some degree of parent participation is expected, I often find myself fully partaking in all of the running, jumping, skipping, and galloping. I know to some, I probably look like a semi-crazed mom hopped up on one too many cups of coffee. For me, it's just another meager attempt to sneak in some physical activity whenever I can. I tell myself that anything and everything is fair game when it comes to burning calories - including buzzing around like a bumblebee!

Aim to exercise four to six days per week for at least thirty to forty minutes at a moderate pace. Try to keep it as fun and varied as you can.

Unless you train competitively either for sport or as a profession, I'm always mindful of activity that appears too strenuous on muscles and joints. Pay attention to your children should they participate in competitive sports. Too much physical strain during adolescence - when ligaments and muscles are still growing - may cause injuries in adulthood that are irreparable. Some of the most physically demanding sports for children include ice hockey, gymnastics, football, and martial arts. However, all sports - if played competitively enough - present risk. Special attention needs to be given for proper rest and adequate recovery from injuries.

Most professional athletes retire young because of the constant physical stress that their bodies have underwent. Bodies are meant to move and stay active, but not put be through the ringer time and time again. Push yourself within reason, but listen to your muscles and joints if you think they've had enough.

Fitness for Life: Christina's Take-Home Points
By Christina VanSike, owner of Capstone Fitness
Indio, CA

Consistency

Consistency is key when it comes to a fitness. While a new year's resolution or important life event may serve as important motivators, remember that fitness needs to be incorporated in your life long term. If you can't picture yourself doing a routine long term, then it's important to try something different that appeals to you better.

Progression

Remember, don't compare your "chapter one" to someone else's "chapter twenty." If you have very little experience with exercise or

---

fitness, start small and progress your way up or else you will end up either injuring yourself or burning yourself out to the point of quitting.

Strength Training

A myth that us trainers are constantly up against is that women feel that strength training will make them bulky. This notion is actually false. Strength training is something that all women should incorporate into their fitness regimen, especially as we age and lose muscle tone. Remember, testosterone is the main hormone responsible for building muscle size. Men have more testosterone than women. In fact, adult males have testosterone levels that are about seven to eight times greater than females. As a woman, your muscles will not be quadrupling in size unless you're taking steroids, spending multiple hours a day training specifically for that goal, or have crazy genetics.

Progress Measuring

The scale is not the end all, be all to your fitness inspirations. Don't forget to measure your progress by how you feel, how your clothes are fitting, and if you are getting stronger. We recommend to our clients to take progress pictures and take measurements, if you are able to. These are very good tools to see if your routine is working.

Make The Time

Women tend to be over-achievers. We want to take care of the kids, run the house, and work full time - amongst everything else. Fitness sometimes ends up being the last on our to-do list. Sometimes we even feel guilty taking the time away to do it. As a mom of two and a personal trainer, I know how important it is to incorporate exercise into our daily regimen. If we are taking care of our bodies, we will have the physical capacity to care for our other responsibilities and priorities even better.

Day 29

Interfere with your body's natural hormone levels as little as possible

Our bodies are equipped with a complex hormone cascade that is designed like an orchestra. Interfering with one or more hormones through the use of medication can drastically throw our mechanisms off. Synthetic hormones in the form of birth control and hormone replacement therapy also have a laundry list of side effects despite their frequency of prescribing. It almost pains me to present these, because I know what a "catch 22 situation" these drugs fall under. Many young women rely on oral contraceptives when the opportunity of bearing a child just isn't appropriate at the time. Both menopausal and post-menopausal women take to synthetic hormones to help with a wide array of conditions brought on by a decrease in estrogen and progesterone. And yet some other women use synthetic hormones to help with menstrual cramps, reduce symptoms of polycystic ovarian syndrome, or in other various conditions. But the harsh fact is that these "one-size-fits-all" hormones are just not completely safe when our body's own hormone levels constantly fluctuate and are completely unique to us.

Serious side effects of synthetic hormones include increased risk for cardiac disease, breast cancer, stroke, and blood clots. These risks are higher for women over 35 years old, smokers, or those who already have high blood pressure. Another important concern regarding oral contraceptives is its link to depression, as noted by a recent study of more than 1 million Danish women. The study found an increased risk for first use of an antidepressant and first diagnosis of depression among users of hormonal contraception - especially in adolescents aged 15 through 19 years old. Because our hormones play a role in the intricate network of "feel-good" neurotransmitters - like serotonin and dopamine - it is no surprise that our bodies' natural web of cognitive communication becomes altered when hormones are replaced synthetically.

So what do women do when it comes to synthetic hormones? First, evaluate if a synthetic hormone is even necessary at all. If being used for contraception, many other hormone-free methods or combination of methods can be just as effective and carry little to no risk. If pregnancy is not foreseeable in the next three to five years, consider using a copper intrauterine device (IUD). Even hormonal IUDs are theoretically "safer," since the hormones are secreted locally in the uterus and less potential to get in the bloodstream. If "the pill" is chosen, try to limit its duration of use and the amount of hormones taken. It is important not to smoke, keep your blood pressure under control, and give it up if you feel like your mental clarity is becoming a little off. If synthetic hormones are being used for menopausal symptoms, it may be wise to talk to your doctor about "bioidentical hormones." These hormones are made to be an exact match in molecular structure to a woman's body, and can be formulated to fit your unique needs based on hormone level testing. Risks still exist with bioidenticals, but you can start low and see how you feel.

Day 30
Find your place in life and do it well

I saved this pearl for last, because it is the hardest, yet most essential goal for you to live as radiantly as possible. I can tell you from personal experience how stressful it is to wake up every morning and try to get through each day feeling like I should be doing something different, more fulfilling and satisfying to my own desires and attributes. My stress levels were the highest in my career when I focused solely on making money at all costs. Yes, we all need to start somewhere in life. We all need to bide time, put our heads down, and endure some degree of hardship and stress until our goals are achieved. But at some point, you have to consider where you are at in life and why you're doing what you're doing.

Everyone has a purpose and a passion - it's just a matter of paying attention to and pursuing the things that spark your match - whether it be personally or professionally. Doing this is part of the much broader act of *aging gracefully*. With age comes wisdom and the discovery of the things we truly like and dislike. If you find yourself habitually waking up miserable and not looking forward to the day, something is wrong and you need to make a change. Stress should never be an ongoing phenomenon. Recognize your talents, stop working solely for a paycheck, know all of your options, surround yourself with motivating people, and start living the life you want.

It is never too late to make changes. Unhappiness and stress are necessary evils, but not dictators of our lives. If you are scared to make a change, just take action and see what happens. Sometimes life changes occur with even the simplest of acts, such as making a phone call or setting up an appointment for yourself or a loved one. You deserve radiant health and a radiant life, and nothing should hold you back from achieving this.

BALANCING CLEAN LIVING
WITH DRUGS

MEDICATIONS WORK BEST in acute conditions when usage is temporary, but the vast majority of Americans take at least one prescription pill every day for chronic conditions, with many taking three or more. It's an umbrella statement - and one I do not like to make - but, in certain circumstances, many men and women are overmedicated. Our desire for antibiotics has created "superbugs" that have learned how to mutate, survive, and thrive in our bodies. The nonchalant prescribing of opioid pain medications has contributed to an addiction epidemic so widespread that deaths by overdose have quadrupled since 1999. And a reliance on antidepressants and anti-anxiety medications is strong enough that many of us are unable to feel "normal" or cope without them. Less drugs will no doubt lead to cleaner living, but we need the knowledge and resources to help decipher the good and evil of modern day medicating. That's where I'm hoping this chapter comes into play.

We shouldn't wholeheartedly be pointing our fingers at doctors and pharmaceutical companies for medication dependence. In fact, many doctors feel immense pressure to prescribe something - anything -just to please their patients, according to a research article published in *Keystone Physician* by Dr. William Sonnenberg. Often, doctors see a rise in their patient satisfaction scores as long as they comply with their patients' wish for treatment. Depending on the circumstance, this often includes an antibiotic, opioid pain medication, test, or admission. The sad fact is that these patients who dictate their own treatment are among the unhealthiest. Researchers also found that the most "satisfied" patients spent the most money on healthcare and prescription drugs, and were even more likely to die!

I found myself in a similar situation when I recently had strep throat. After finding someone to watch my two little ones and waiting close to 2 hours at an urgent care facility, the rapid strep test that the doctor administered came back negative. Since I just had a mere sore throat, I was sent on my way with instructions to rest up and use ibuprofen. My throat pain was so severe and lymph nodes so swollen, that I was incredulous and couldn't believe my appointment was for naught. In fact, I started to get pretty upset walking out of the clinic empty handed, even though I knew my condition didn't currently warrant the use of an antibiotic. I even called my husband and sobbed that I just wasted 2 and 1/2 hours sitting around, and I could've been doing anything else since I was sans kids - errands, working, or just trying to get better! I should probably mention this incident was shortly after my second son was born, so the sleep deprivation was probably getting the best of me at this point!

The moral of my story is that I ended up being upset at the clinic for not giving me an antibiotic, even though I knew so much better. Both society and the essence of human nature want us to seek resolution if there is ever a problem, so I think this is why so many of us desire treatment in the form of medication when our health goes awry. When we walk out of the doctor's office with a script in hand, it validates our effort in a sense and gives us a tangible declaration that we are working towards fixing our condition. Going back to my strep throat story, my throat swab was eventually sent to a lab for more sensitive testing. I did, indeed, have strep throat and felt 100% better with some amoxicillin and prednisone.

My strep throat story - albeit simple in terms of health issues - only supports my claim that I am not against medications. For acute conditions, terminal illnesses, and chronic conditions that have failed other therapies, pharmaceuticals are often at the crux of our health.

I do have to mention that I've seen a large progression towards the "all-natural" way and have seen people get into major trouble. I've witnessed children's illnesses never resolve due to the parents' hesitation to bring them to the doctor or reluctance to give them a medication. It doesn't take long for them to see that the "holistic" recipe they found on a website is not working, and now their child's fever, stomach ache, or whatever other ailment is getting worse by the day. This "100% drug-free" progression is yet another extreme swing of the pendulum that can put people in grave danger.

Every single day, I see articles written or medical products endorsed - or even created - by people with all different types of backgrounds. For everyday health, these sources are perfectly fine. However, for the vast majority of decisions, you should always consult a professional who not only understands the statistics, but your own personal history and concerns. While a mere passion for wellness speaks volumes, it does not make up the many years, devotion, and intense work that constitutes a medical degree. People who pursue these degrees and acquire the necessary experience go through ringer simply because this field requires nothing less.

I sense that if the extreme, all-natural progression continues, the desired effect will be opposite and potentially even detrimental to our society. Again, balance is key. Medications are not "bad," but they need to be used properly. It is imperative to find a trusted professional who not only has the knowledge, but the *clinical experience* to help guide you and your family.

If you do find yourself seeking information online, try to limit your perusing to sites that are created or backed by professionals. I really like taking recommendations from the U.S. Task Force, which is made up of a group of volunteer doctors and other professionals who sift through all of the data. If I read from another website, I try to look for listed references that mention where the writers or researchers obtained their information. References such as studies, books, educational seminars, or other reputable websites are all valid and give the article much more substance.

Leave Well Enough Alone

Through my years of clinical practice, I've learned that sometimes it is best to let sleeping dogs lie, in a sense. I first experienced this notion as a young intern and have seen countless cases since then. If a routine or regimen is working, then let it be.

When I was still in pharmacy school, I did an internship at a local hospital. An older physician worked there whom I admired and whose opinion I always sought. He was a "cool" doctor, with his prominent glasses, Hawaiian floral shirts, and khaki shorts. In fact, his white coat was often longer than his shorts, so it sort of gave the appearance that he wasn't wearing anything underneath if you happened to catch the backside of him. Thinking about him wandering the hospital halls appearing half-naked still makes me chuckle. He was a pretty special doctor.

One morning, I found myself doing rounds with him and a handful of other healthcare professionals. An elderly woman had been admitted the night before, and we were busy looking over her history and medication profile.

One younger doctor noticed that she had been taking the medication, amitriptyline. Amitriptyline is an older generation antidepressant that can also be used for various other reasons. The young doctor chirped up and stated, "We should definitely discontinue her amitriptyline. It's on the Beer's Criteria, and she's over 65 years old."

The Beer's Criteria is a list of drugs that are deemed hazardous for the elderly. Because amitriptyline is very sedating and can put the elderly population at risk for falls, it is very rarely recommended for those over 65 years old. For all intents and purposes, this young doctor was on point.

Finally! I thought to myself, because I, too, had noticed this woman was on amitriptyline and, at last, felt the pieces of my education coming together. Pharmacists are trained to see these red flags, and I was proud of myself for catching this.

However, the other doctor - the one with the shorts - said something unexpected that threw me off guard. He stated something to this effect, "Discontinuing her amitriptyline is actually one of the last things I would do at this point. She's been taking this medication for twenty-some odd years. She reports feeling good on it and has become tolerant to the side effects. Why rock the boat just because the literature tells us to? Experience tells me otherwise."

Needless to say, the whole team agreed to keep her on the medication with extra monitoring of her vital organs.

Fast forward years later, and I still remind myself of this scenario whenever someone asks about wanting to discontinue a medication. Now, certain circumstances do apply here, and sometimes I'm very much on board to discontinue a medication, or at least attempt a trial of discontinuation. Other times, I'm apt to leave well enough alone. So long as the drug is still safe and working, why disrupt an effective regimen? Again, this is up to you and your doctor to decide.

Medication Misuse and Abuse

Today's world affords us the luxury of blending cutting edge medical research with ancient modalities to live the life we want. What I am against is the abuse of medications, and this can occur in several ways:

Polypharmacy

This term refers to the use of multiple medications to treat one or more conditions. Sometimes this is required, but toxicities arise when mistakes are made with this type of regimen. Mistakes such as using multiple medications from a similar drug class or not maxing out a dose of a medication before another one is added are very common. I once saw three of the same types of blood pressure medication on a patient's profile. Apparently, the elderly woman had seen a second doctor to get another opinion, but failed to mention to this doctor what she was already taking. The doctor unknowingly prescribed her something very similar to an existing drug, yet she later went on to experience side effects. She returned to the same doctor who then gave her a prescription for another drug in a similar class in an effort to thwart the side effects. Meanwhile, she never stopped taking anything and was inadvertently using three different medications that worked the same way. It was very easy for her to get confused, and the miscommunication led to a polypharmacy situation which could have been incredibly dangerous for her.

If a medication regimen can be streamlined, the safer and easier it will be for everyone involved. The more drugs that are added to the mix, the more likely for interactions and side effects to pile up and cause toxicities. In many circumstances, our bodies just simply cannot absorb multiple medications. When inundated with a lot of exogenous chemicals, consider it "overload" for our internal network.

The cells in our bodies can only process so many chemicals at once. If our liver and kidneys are overburdened with processing alcohol, drugs, or toxic substances, it simply cannot keep up.

As a side note, this is precisely why I decided to delay the MMR vaccine in my children. Although routinely given at one year of age and regarded as safe, I just wasn't completely confident that such a young immune system could safely handle and process a triple live vaccine. In many other parts of the world, vaccines - whether live or inactivated - are delayed until 2 years of age, when the immune system has matured enough to handle them. Childhood vaccines are controversial and outside of the realm of this book. However, if you are interested, I recommend referencing the works of Dr. William Sears. I will say this: I am in favor of childhood vaccinations, but I do recommend looking into a partially delayed approach and never giving more than three or four vaccines at a time in order to not overload a child's young system. Actually, a very counterintuitive fact is that most vaccines provide better coverage if more time is allowed between them.

If a baby is not in daycare, some vaccines, such as the rotavirus, can be waived completely. However, if you and your baby travel a lot - even within the country - I can only recommend adhering to the standard vaccination schedule. Different geographical locations are exposed to different strains of bacteria and viruses, which your child's young immune system may not be able to recognize and fight. Only vaccinations can protect your child.

Especially if your child has an illness, you need to have a frank discussion with your pediatrician to determine the safest vaccination schedule. We all have an ethical responsibility to protect our children in the safest way possible.

Returning to adults, you'd be surprised how many terminally ill patients with complicated regimens that I've actually seen improve when a "drug holiday" was taken. Given the opportunity to discontinue most, if not all, medications is highly dependent on many variables (remember, these men and women only had months left to live) - but doing so may allow the body to start transmitting and processing information more effectively without the chemical disruption of pharmaceuticals. The system's natural tendency to restore homeostasis returns, and people report feeling better, less tired or "fuzzy", and generally more enhanced. Medications can then be reintroduced on the basis of necessity.

Prescription cascade

As a general rule of thumb, never use another medication to treat the side effects from the original drug. An example of prescription cascade would be using an antianxiety medication to treat the side effect of anxiety caused by an antidepressant. Unless in the case of panic attacks, an antianxiety medication and antidepressant should rarely ever be taken together. Antianxiety medications have a "depressing" effect, which is intended to calm down the nervous system. These medications can actually make depression worse and cause a vicious cycle in which the user of both medications never really gets better.

This is why it is very important to know the most common side effects of a medication, so, in the event of an undesirable side effect, every effort can be made to either lower the dose or switch to another medication with a more favorable side effect profile.

Antidepressants: The Good, the Bad, and During Pregnancy

Many experts believe that antidepressants are overprescribed. What's more concerning are the opinions surrounding how effective antidepressants actually are. The range of these opinions is uncomfortably vast, spanning from "not effective at all" to "essential." My view on antidepressants is unfortunately a little fuzzy as well and tends to lie somewhere in between. I have seen many a script for these coveted drugs presented to the pharmacy and can't help but wonder if they are indeed overly prescribed, and if they are actually helping my patients. The medical community has set out to analyze these observations as well, and many studies and essays exist in effort to shed some light. While the opinions vary on overutilization and efficacy, the consensus seems to agree on one thing - approach antidepressants with caution.

Studies show that the benefit of antidepressants is highly dependent on the severity of the depression. They probably don't work that well - if at all - in mild depression, but could be highly effective in severe depression. One issue is the length of time it takes for an antidepressant to start working. Generally speaking, it can take a long time for the benefits to start kicking in, but the side effects are often felt right away. Over half of all people using antidepressants report side effects such as dry mouth, headaches, digestion problems, feeling faint or anxious, and decreased sex drive. Various studies also suggest that teenagers consider suicide more often when taking an antidepressant and also actually attempt suicide more often. It is important to ask yourself if the possible benefits of the antidepressant outweigh these potential side effects and dangers.

What I personally find the most concerning, however, is the sometimes impossible task of finding the right antidepressant or combination of antidepressants that actually work for the patient. This notion has led to a onslaught of various new medications whose sole purpose is to "help" an existing antidepressant work better or to target depression by a different mechanism. This is because many people fail to getter with the drug that is originally prescribed to them, and sometimes even fail second and third options as well. In the meantime, they are still dealing with the depression on a daily basis, may even be experiencing side effects of the drug, and wasting money on the copays. Relying on the drug to work, they may not choose to seek other ways to get better, such as counseling or behavioral therapy. Drug therapy is highly personalized, and the many months it can take to get it just right can be frustrating and downright futile.

It is also important to remember that antidepressants only work if there is a *neurochemical* imbalance - in other words, serotonin, dopamine, and other "feel good" neurotransmitters are quantifiably lower than average. If your low mood is not due to a chemical imbalance, antidepressants will not work for you.

Studies also show a huge "placebo effect" when studying antidepressants. People report that they are getting better even if they are taking a placebo, simply because they feel as if whatever they are taking should be helping. Other studies have found that counseling or other therapies - such as meditation or exercise - work even better than drugs in treating depression, but are often not presented or offered to those who suffer.

Lastly, if you are pregnant or thinking of becoming pregnant, antidepressants should be the absolute last resort to treat depression. I know what you are thinking, and I agree - antidepressant use during pregnancy is a hugely controversial, yet individualized issue whose risks and benefits need to be weighed against your own personal situation. All you need to do is type the keywords into any search engine, and a slew of articles and studies emerge that sometimes only add to the confusion. All of these studies help to shed some light, but no one really knows how a drug will work with your own (and your baby's) chemistry.

Know this - given the amount of alternative therapies that exist to treat depression, exhaust them first. Some of the neurotransmitters that antidepressants work on have the potential to affect the baby's nervous system and cognitive development while in utero. Using antidepressants during pregnancy has also been associated with preterm birth - a situation that presents its own problems, regardless of antidepressant use. The risks are real enough to consider going to great lengths to find alternate therapy. By great lengths, I mean using a multi-modality approach and giving each therapy an adequate chance to work. Counseling, meditation, yoga, light therapy, acupuncture, pet therapy, spirituality, and volunteering are all valid non-drug ways to combat depression.

However, if the stress of depression is more of a risk to the baby than the actual antidepressant, then know that many studies have had positive or neutral results with most of the newer medications. As with almost every other medication for any other condition, "start low and go slow."

If you are already using an antidepressant and become pregnant, try to slowly wean off the medication and see how you do. You may even be able to lower the dose in an effort to decrease exposure. Remember that medications may affect you and your baby differently according to the trimester. The first trimester is a time for exponential growth of the baby's brain. If you can, it is best to avoid chemicals and unnecessary medications during this time.

Given all the uncertainty and side effects surrounding antidepressants, it only makes sense to second guess the drugs that are commonly prescribed. If you are experiencing depression due to a transient event in life, such as divorce or death, consider the potential time and treatment failures that it could take to actually receive benefit from a drug. Time - with or without pharmaceutical intervention - can heal a lot on its own. On the other hand, severe depression should be diagnosed and treated properly. Antidepressants do have a place in therapy here and can truly help people cope in everyday life or give them the impetus to seek other forms of help.

Taking a drug with no established benefit

This seems pretty self-explanatory, but many people take medications without any substantial evidence backing its use or no condition that warrants it. I used to see this example a lot back when certain antacid medications, called proton-pump inhibitors, were frequently prescribed for stress ulcer prevention in patients with long hospital stays. The most common one was Prilosec, or omeprazole. After the illness resolved, the patient would eventually be discharged from the hospital with their list of medications. The problem is that omeprazole would still be on the medication profile. Sometimes, months or even years would go by and they would still be taking this medication, even though their risk for developing a stress ulcer was long gone. No one really thought to ask about it or discontinue it.

A one-size-fits-all approach

Western medicine relies almost exclusively on information gained from clinical trials, which are studies that are conducted in large groups of people to either research a new cure or ascertain better treatment options using preexisting therapies. These trials are the backbone that support the drugs that are frequently prescribed and can provide useful information for clinicians when faced with uncertainty. The problem with these trials is that they often utilize specific "inclusion and exclusion criteria" when it comes to selecting the group of people that will be participating in the study. Both pregnant and non-pregnant women, minorities, young adults and children, the elderly, and people who have other problematic disease states are among those that are often underrepresented in clinical trials.

The researchers of the study may exclude certain populations for a couple of reasons. Firstly, studying a more homogenous population makes for a smoother evaluation and gathering of results, especially the results they have in mind and are hoping to achieve. Secondly, safety and ethical concerns can have huge implications if not carefully weighed. This is often why pregnant women, children, and those with disease states or conditions that make it difficult to find a safe dose are usually excluded in clinical trials. It is just too easy for these patients to be at risk for harm. And, generally speaking, the more diverse a patient population is, the harder it is to account for all the different scenarios that can go wrong. Too many factors can negate the vast effort put in to conducting a useful study.

So we know that some exclusion criteria is absolutely necessary, however the extent of which patients are left out of the study can make it hard to apply the results to the general population. The "general population" are the people like you and me - with diverse backgrounds and different states of health - that show up to the doctor's office and receive the same drug with the same dose and same expectation of response.

Even other factors in clinical trials such as the setting, the ease of the medication regimen, and the types of statistical tests used to evaluate the data can all contribute to how well - or not well - the results can be applied to everyday clinical practice. This is how prescribing based on results from trials - which may not adequately portray the most realistic scenario - can lead to a one-size-fits-all approach in which the average population will undoubtedly experience an array of reactions, side effects, and degrees of tolerability to the same studied regimen. You probably have seen the myriad of legal advertisements offering large settlements to those afflicted by severe side effects - years after the medication had been approved and established in the "real world," when such information was eventually brought to light.

The good news is that many clinicians are aware of the one-size-fits-all approach and do their best to circumvent the problem. Issues such as age, organ function, gender, other preexisting disease states, drug interactions, and even drug-food interactions should all be taken into account before selecting an appropriate medication and dose. These factors are all highly individualized and can affect the way we respond to a certain medication.

Going even one step further, cutting research in a field called *pharmacogenomics* is continuously taking place. This field studies how a person's genes can affect their response to a particular drug. You could look at it as "tailored" therapy, cut specifically to your genetic makeup. Antidepressants are just one group of medications that are being studied as personalized therapy. Several genes have been identified that may play a role in how well someone responds to a group of antidepressants called SSRIs - selective seratonin reuptake inhibitors. A greater response to the medication may prevent relapses in depression and may also cut down on side effects by utilizing more appropriate therapy at a potentially lower dose. Another drug that has high implications in pharmacogenomics is the popular and often dangerous blood thinner, warfarin. A genetic test - which isn't routinely done yet - can be conducted before warfarin is started and can dictate a safer dose. Further research and cost-effectiveness studies are needed before personalized therapy can create a niche for itself in modern day medicine. However, you can see the many individualized factors that go into play when medications are introduced.

Polypharmacy, prescription cascade, and one-size-fits-all approach are just a few examples that demonstrate how easy it is for drugs to complicate a clean lifestyle. Knowledge and prevention of these errors can often impede a vicious cycle in which drugs accumulate, interactions build, and side effects impinge on the essence of daily living. Much of this awareness and empowerment begins in the doctor's office. This can be difficult though, because the office setting is somewhat uncomfortable for many people and not ideal for more comprehensive inquiring about symptoms or treatment. You may feel rushed. You may be wondering why he or she is prescribing a particular medication based on the symptoms you presented. You may even feel powerless, no matter how empathetic and compassionate your care provider may be.

> *Remember, knowledge is a powerful weapon against uncertainty.*

The Hippocratic oath states that clinicians have a "special obligation to all fellow human beings." The population they serve is undeniably their utmost priority. But, despite the trust and faith we put in our doctors and other professionals, the ultimate responsibility and ownership of optimal health lies within you. A basic knowledge of the treatment process, especially YOUR treatment process, is crucial before any pill is ingested or test scanned. A cleaner life can start with a cleaner medicine cabinet and the ability to take charge of your health.

Try to remember to ask these important questions the next time you find yourself in the passenger's seat at the doctor's office.

Is a drug really necessary for my condition?

Don't be afraid to ask your doctor about possible nondrug options and the consequences of going without the drug. Take depression again for example, a condition that affects nearly every one of us at one time or another. Many times, other nondrug therapy such as counseling, exercise, acupuncture, and even pet therapy work substantially better than some of the most common antidepressants prescribed - and without the side effects. As previously mentioned, depression is also considered an episodic illness, which is something that is often precipitated by a life event. Once the issue resolves, the depression may lift - yet many antidepressants are prescribed indefinitely and never discontinued. This continuous prescribing often puts people in a position where they feel dependent on the drug and lose their ability to cope without it.

Many also suffer from low back pain and find themselves reaching for over-the-counter pain relievers or stronger, yet potentially more dangerous prescription analgesics. However, recommendations from the American College of Physicians urges both physicians and patients to skip drug therapy as a first-line treatment for acute back pain. They note that alternative therapies such as massage, acupuncture, chiropractic treatment, and yoga are all viable and potentially more effective options that should be exhausted first. Surprisingly, the evidence from these recommendations shows that acctaminophen treatment was no more effective than placebo in improving back pain, even though it is frequently used. And opioid medications, like hydrocodone and oxycodone, should be considered only as a last resort after everything else has failed. Opioids should be considered a last resort for all types of pain - not just back pain - so be wary if any practitioner is quick to prescribe them.

If a doctor is prescribing a brand new drug that recently hit the market (I talk about this more in a later section) or is suggesting preventative therapy (such as for high blood pressure or cholesterol), ask about something called the NNT or "number needed to treat." Going back to clinical trials, the NNT is a statistical calculation that refers to the number of people you need to treat in order for one person to have a positive outcome. Basically, it measures the effectiveness of the drug therapy. You want the NNT to be very low - essentially one - which would mean that every person treated improves. Many of us perceive modern medicine in this fashion -

those who are treated derive benefit, whereas those who are not treated don't.

The NNT is often higher than what we like to see, which means the drug in question may not be all that effective. When clinicians are aware of the NNT, they tend to make more conservative decisions regarding drug therapy. If a doctor doesn't know the NNT associated with a new drug and fails to look it up for you, don't take stock in the prescription.

Sometimes, we may experience a minor condition that puts us in the pharmacy aisle instead of in a doctor's office. You can ask yourself or your pharmacist the same question about possible non-drug therapies. Probiotics for a child's constipation, epsom salts for muscle or joint pain, and hydration for headaches are just a few examples of minor, often isolated situations that don't require drugs.

How exactly does this drug work and when will I see benefit?

Know exactly what to expect from your medication and be realistic about all possible outcomes. Many people are unaware that antidepressants generally take three to four weeks to see therapeutic benefit, however most will experience side effects during that time. Not knowing when a drug will start to work may lead to early discontinuation, unnecessary dosage increases, or the addition of another drug which may be less appropriate. How long the treatment will last and how refills are handled should be also be discussed.

What are the most common adverse effects?

Your doctor or pharmacist should be ready and willing to discuss all possible side effects, interactions (including food and supplement interactions), allergies, and possible activities to avoid while taking the medication. Knowing the common risks can save a lot of unnecessary trouble and even dangerous events. For example, some antibiotics can make skin extra sensitive to sunlight and cause extreme sunburns or rashes. Wearing a higher SPF, protective clothing, and staying out of direct sunlight while on the medication can prevent the discomfort and danger of a sunburn. The discussion of avoidable activities and interactions are often neglected. Knowing what to do should an adverse event occur is also important.

If the doctor is prescribing more than one drug to treat the same condition, what is the reason behind this?

Some drugs work synergistically together, meaning that the combined effect from both medications is greater than from one single agent. Other times - especially for some refractory conditions that don't respond well to just one drug - another drug from a different class is added to the regimen. If your doctor is prescribing in a synergistic fashion or is using multiple drugs for better targeting, he or she needs to explain this to you. A multiple drug regimen is occasionally needed for some situations. However, more times than not, multiple drugs for the same illness or condition just mean more potential for side effects and interactions. If you feel your condition is not being adequately treated, always check to see that your medication's dose is appropriately maxed out before adding another. And if you've seen more than one physician to treat the same problem, ensure that they are all aware of what you've already been prescribed and that old drugs are discontinued.

If the doctor is prescribing a brand new drug that recently became approved, what qualities about the drug or my condition warrant this?

For a brand new drug to hit the market, it would have went through a series of clinical trials to study the safety, tolerance, optimum dosage, and side effects. The drug is first studied in animals, then eventually makes its way up to humans. By the time the drug hits the last study - or Phase III clinical trial - the drug is tested on a large scale to verify its effectiveness and to establish long term safety. A Phase III trial is good news for a drug; if it made it this far and does well here, the chances of it getting approved and being prescribed to the general population are extremely high. And the drug company can finally start cashing in on some "cha-ching" for all the work they put out.

However, one cannot assume that a drug is completely safe if it passes a Phase III trial and gets approved. First, it is important to be aware of a possible bias in which only "positive" results are reported from the studies. Drug companies are faced with two immense pressures to have a drug live up to its claim - time and money. Companies often fund their own studies, since no one else will. Also, a drug only has a twenty year patent from the time it was invented. Considering the many years of research involved before a drug can make it to Phase III, twenty years is not a long time before copycats can emerge. Couple the financial implications with a ticking time bomb patent, and the situation becomes stressful for many companies.

Many factors have to be considered when evaluating a clinical trial. Awareness of the tendency for researchers and drug companies to publish only the good stuff is crucial. No study can be free of bias. Even though complicated statistical tests are used to evaluate their results, these are often hard to interpret and assess for appropriateness. It can also be easy to skew the numbers in an effort to exaggerate a claim. After all, a drug is supposed to work, and the data needs to show this in order for doctors to start prescribing it. Remember the all-important NNT and make sure your doctor is aware of it. Returning to our "one-size-fits-all" discussion, bear in mind that clinical trials often have specific inclusion criteria and are conducted in settings that don't always accurately represent real-life scenarios.

Considering these issues, it's no surprise that a keen and unbiased eye is required to critically evaluate a new drug and to weed out all the fluff. My job is not to throw pharmaceutical companies under the bus, but to introduce the unglamorous factors that their marketing department tries so diligently to offset. Glossy advertisements with attractive actors spark our interest more than we like to admit. But you have every right to be wary about brand new drugs and deserve to know all the reasons why it may or may not be appropriate for you.

Drug use - whether prescription or over the counter, legal or recreational - is undeniably one of the most significant considerations when it comes to radiant health. Even the most benign of medications can be potentially toxic and wreak havoc on a healthy individual if used inappropriately.

Exogenous chemicals affect the delicate and intricate internal networks that our bodies have fine-tuned throughout all of our evolution, whether this mechanism is part of the intended result or not.

Needless to say, we all will inevitably still reach for the pill vial at one point or another. Hopefully, armed with some of this knowledge, you can start taking the first steps in evaluating whether or not some medications are really necessary for your health and lifestyle and how to use them safely and effectively if they are.

A Final Word

I HOPE YOU'VE enjoyed reading this book as much as I've enjoyed writing it. This "final word" finds me with two young children at home and motherhood still relatively new to me in the grand scheme of things. My purpose for writing this book was two-fold - to not only share the knowledge I've acquired as a healthcare professional throughout the years, but to remind myself of the daily habits that I personally need to practice for both myself and my young family. At the end of the day, my goal is to be able to see my grown children happy and partaking in life. I personally want to enjoy every other aspect of life, too. Your situation may be near or far from mine, but the lessons of devoting time and energy to your health still apply.

More importantly, I hope you feel *empowered* to take charge of your health and life. While your genes can make you susceptible to a boatload of conditions, it is ultimately your habits that decipher your health and the path in life you choose to take. It really does take only thirty days - and sometimes even less - for drastic mind and body improvement.

Remember, everything starts with your mind. Perception is everything, and especially the way you perceive yourself. Staying optimistic and focusing on the quality of your life will undeniably keep you feeling young and healthy, no matter what age you are.

Also remember that your needs and priorities will change as you age and encounter different life circumstances. You don't have the same body you did as a child, nor will you have the same body years from now. You will be exposed to different environments, different stresses, and hormonal changes as you age. Writing this book also reminds me that every stage, every situation in a woman's life is temporary. Not only are we highly dynamic creatures, but the world we live in changes around us as well.

No matter the situation or stage in life you're in, keep your health a top priority. Always keep the basics in mind, like proper sleep and nutrition. The basics will save you from spending time, energy, and money on unnecessary medications and artificial beauty regimens in the long run. The basics will also allow you to keep your sanity in a culture that's inundated with new products, advertisements, and endorsements.

Remember to nurture your relationships. Focus on the people in your life, and not your things. Having nice things only create a temporary fulfillment; your relationships (including the one you have with yourself) will establish lifelong happiness. Take pride in yourself and your life; true radiance will follow.

References

1. Lantz, G. (2014, February 27). Brain Differences Between Genders. *Psychology Today*. Retrieved from www.psychologytoday.com

2. Kanazawa, S. (2008, March 17). Male Brain vs. Female Brain. *Pyschology today*. Retrieved from www.psychologytoday. com

3. Hakim, R. B., et al. "Alcohol and caffeine consumption and decreased fertility." *Fertility and Sterility* Volume 70, no. 4 (1998): 632-637.

4. Westphal, L.W., et al. "A nutritional supplement for improving fertility in women." *The Journal of Reproductive Medicine*. Volume 49, no. 4 (2004): 289-293.

5. Linehan, M. (1993). *Skills training manual for treating borderline personality disorder*. New York, NY: Guilford Press.

6. Scott, J. (2014). *At home with madame chic*. New York, NY: Simon & Schuster.

7. Shannon, Joseph. "Changing How We Feel by Changing How We Think." Cumberland County College, Vineland. 2 May 1017. Lecture.

8. Harvey, J. (2016, November 2). French mothers don't suffer from bladder incontinence. And nor should you. *The Guardian*. Retrieved from www.theguardian.com

9. Katayose Y, et al. Carryover effect on next-day sleepiness and psychomotor performance of nighttime administered antihistaminic drugs: A randomized controlled trial. *Human Psychopharmacology Clinical and Experimental*. 2012;27:428.

10. Side effects of sleep drugs. U.S. Food and Drug Administration. http://www.fda.gov/ForConsumers/ConsumerUpdates/ucm107757.htm#otc

11. Gray SL, et al. Cumulative use of strong anticholinergics and incident dementia: A prospective cohort study. *JAMA Internal Medicine*. 2015;175:401.

12. Carriere I, et al. Drugs with anticholinergic properties, cognitive decline, and dementia in an elderly general population: The 3-city study. *Archives of Internal Medicine*. 2009;169:1317

13. "Alcohol Alert," *National Institute on Alcohol Abuse and Alcoholism*. October 2004, accessed from https://pubs.niaaa.nih.gov/publications/aa63/aa63.htm

14. Mercola, J. (2017). Fluoridated water destroys your brain and teeth. *Mercola*. Retrieved from www.articles.mercola.com

15. Hood, Ernie. The Apple Bites Back: Claiming Old Orchards for Residential Development. *Environmental Health Perspectives*. 2006 Aug; 114(8): A470–A476.

16. Sambrook P, Cooper C. Osteoporosis. *Lancet*. 2006; 367:2010–2018.

17. Gerdhem P, Ringsberg KA, Obrant KJ, Akesson K. Association between 25-hydroxy vitamin D levels, physical activity, muscle strength and fractures in the prospective population-based OPRA Study of Elderly Women. *Osteoporosis Int*. 2005;16:1425–1431.

18. Mithal, A., Wahl, D.A., Bonjour, JP. et al. Global vitamin D status and determinants of hypovitaminosis D. *Osteoporos Int* (2009) 20: 1807.

19. Holick M (2002) Vitamin D: the underappreciated D-lightful hormone that is important for skeletal and cellular health. *Curr Opin Endocrinol Diabetes Obes* 9:87–98

20. Holick MF (1999) Evolution, biologic functions, and recommended dietary allowance for vitamin D. In: Holick MF (ed) Vitamin D: physiology, molecular biology and clinical applications. Humana Press, Totowa, New Jersey, pp 1–16

21. Susan M. Ott; Long-Term Safety of Bisphosphonates. *J Clin Endocrinol Metab* 2005; 90 (3): 1897-1899.

22. Whyte, M. P., McAlister, W. H., Novack, D. V., Clements, K. L., Schoenecker, P. L. and Wenkert, D. (2008), Bisphosphonate-Induced Osteopetrosis: Novel Bone Modeling Defects, Metaphyseal Osteopenia, and Osteosclerosis Fractures After Drug Exposure Ceases. *J Bone Miner Res*, 23: 1698–1707

23. Sunscreens/sunblocks. The American Academy of Dermatology Web site. www.aad.org/public/publications/pamphlets/sun_sunscreens.html.

24. Crosby K. Prevention of sun-induced skin disorders. In: Berardi

R, Newton G, McDermott JH, et al, eds. *Handbook of Nonprescription Drugs.* 16th ed. Washington, DC: American Pharmacists Association; 2009:729-733.

25. Chen, W. Y., et al. "Moderate alcohol consumption during adult life, drinking patterns, and breast cancer risk." *JAMA* 306, no.17 (2011): 1884-90.

26. Choonipicharn, S., et al. "Antioxidant and antihypertensive activity of gelatin hydrolysate from Nile tilapia skin." *Journal of Food Science and Technology* 52, no. 5 (2014): 3134-39; Ao, J., et al. "Amino acid composition and antioxidant activities of hydrolysates and peptide fractions from porcine collagen." *Food Science and Technology International* 18, no. 5 (2012): 425-34.

27. Leem, K. H., et al. "Porcine skin gelatin hydrolysate promotes longitudinal bone growth in adolescent rats." *Journal of Medicinal Food* 16, no. 5 (1013): 447-53.

28. Friedlander, B. "New York red wines show higher levels of resveratrol, a Cornell University study finds." *Cornell Chronicle*, February 2, 1998.

29. Rollison, D.E., et al. "Personal hair dye use and cancer: a systematic literature review and evaluation of exposure assessment in studies published since 1992." *Journal of Toxicology and Environmental Health, Part B* 9, no. 5 (2006): 413-19

30. Heikkinen, S., et al. "Does hair dye use increase the risk of breast cancer? A population based case-control study of Finnish women." *PloS* One 10, no. 8 (2015)

31. Toich, Laurie. (2017, June 21). FDA Warns of Body Building Supplements Containing Steroids. *The American Journal of Pharmacy Benefits.* Retrieved from http://www.ajpb.com/news/fda-warns-of-body-building-supplements-containing-steroids

32. Thomas, Mathilde. (2015). *The French Beauty Solution: Time Tested Secrets to Look and Feel Beautiful Inside and Out.* New York, NY: Penguin Random House.

33. Vieira, A., et al. "The Role of Probiotics and Prebiotics in Inducing Gut Immunity." *Frontiers in Immunology*, no. 4 (2013).

34. Yan, F., et al. "Probiotics and immune health." Current Opinion in Gastroenterology, 27 (6):496-501. (2011)

35. Janeway, CA Jr., et al. The immune system in health and disease. *Immunobiology*, 5th edition. New York, NY: Garland Science (2001)

36. Skovlund CW, Mørch LS, Kessing LV, et al. Association of Hormonal Contraception With Depression. *JAMA Psychiatry*, Published online September 28 2016

37. Sonnenberg, William MD. Patient Satisfaction is Overrated. *Keystone Physician*, a publication of the Pennsylvania Academy of Family Physicians. Fall 2013.

38. Santarsieri, D., et al. Antidepressant efficacy and side effect burden: a quick guide for clinicians. *Drugs in Context*, 4: 212290. (2015)

39. Tuccori, M., et al. Safety concerns associated with the use of serotonin reuptake inhibitors and other serotonergic/noradrenergic antidepressants during pregnancy: A review. *Clinical Therapeutics*, Volume 31, Part 1, 2009, pages 1426-1453

40. Tsourounis, Candy. How to Evaluate a Randomized Controlled Trial: What Every Pharmacist Should Know. *Hospital Pharmacy*, Volume 35, no. 10: 1071-1078

41. Schulz, Kenneth. Subverting Randomization in Controlled Trials. *JAMA*, Volume 274, no. 18 (1995)

42. Kendrach, M., et al. Calculating Risks and Number-Needed-to-Treat: A Method of Data Interpretation. *Journal of Managed Care Pharmacy*, Volume 3, no. 2 (1997)

43. Qaseem, A., et al. Noninvasive Treatments for Acute, Subacute, and Chronic Low Back Pain: A Clinical Practice Guideline From the American College of Physicians. Annals of Internal Medicine. 2017: 166 (7): 514-530

44. Yang, A., et al. Neonatal discontinuation syndrome in serotonergic antidepressant-exposed neonates. *Journal of Clinical Psychiatry*, 2017;78(5):605–611

45. Committee to Review Dietary Reference Intakes for Vitamin D and Calcium, Food and Nutrition Board, Institute of Medicine. Dietary Reference Intakes for Calcium and Vitamin D. Washington, DC: National Academy Press, 2010

46. National Institutes of Health. Optimal calcium intake. NIH Consensus Statement: 1994;12:1-31.

47. Gao X, LaValley MP, Tucker KL. Prospective studies of dairy product and calcium intakes and prostate cancer risk: a meta-analysis. *J Natl Cancer Inst.* 2005;97:1768-1777.

48. Weingarten MA, Zalmanovici A, Yaphe J. Dietary calcium supplementation for preventing colorectal cancer and adenomatous polyps. Cochrane Database Syst Rev. 2008 Jan 23;(1):CD003548.

49. Michaelsson K, Melhus H, Warensjo Lemming E, Wold A, Byberg L. Long term calcium intake and rates of all cause and cardiovascular mortality: community based prospective longitudinal cohort study. *BMJ* 2013;12;346:f228

50. Bolland MJ, Avenell A, Baron JA, Grey A, MacLennan GS, Gamble GD, Reid IR.Effect of calcium supplements on risk of myocardial infarction and cardiovascular events: meta-analysis. *BMJ.* 2010 Jul 29;341:c3691.

51. Bolland MJ, Barber PA, Doughty RN, Mason B, Horne A, Ames R, Gamble GD, Grey A, Reid IR. Vascular events in healthy older women receiving calcium supplementation: randomised controlled trial. *BMJ.* 2008; 2;336:262-266

52. Li K, Kaaks R, Linseisen J, Rohrmann S. Associations of dietary calcium intake and calcium supplementation with myocardial infarction and stroke risk and overall cardiovascular mortality in the Heidelberg cohort of the European Prospective Investigation into Cancer and Nutrition study (EPIC-Heidelberg). *Heart.* 2012;98:920-925.

53. Xiao Q, Murphy RA, Houston DK, Harris TB, Chow WH, Park Y. Dietary and Supplemental Calcium Intake and Cardiovascular Disease Mortality: The National Institutes of Health-AARP Diet and Health Study. *JAMA Intern Med.* 2013 Feb 4:1-8.

54. Wang L, Manson JE, Sesso HD. Calcium intake and risk of cardiovascular disease: a review of prospective studies and randomized clinical trials. *Am J Cardiovasc Drugs* 2012;12:105-16

55. Conte, J. M., & Jacobs, R. R. (2003). Validity evidence linking polychronicity and Big 5 personality dimensions to absence, lateness, and performance. *Human Performance*, 16, 107-129.

56. Vera-Villarroel, P., et al. Analysis of the relationship between the Type A behavior pattern and fear of negative evaluation. *International Journal of Clinical Health and Psychology*. 2004, Vol. 4, no.2, 313-322.

57. Siska, Gunda. Why I do NOT routinely recommend calcium supplements to maintain strong bones. *Pharmacy Times*. April 19, 2017

58. WHO recommendations for prevention and treatment of pre-eclampsia and eclampsia. Geneva: World Health Organization; 2011 (http://www.who.int/reproductivehealth/publications/maternal_per inatal_health/9789241548335/en/)

59. Guideline: Calcium supplementation in pregnant women. Geneva: World Health Organization; 2013 (http://www.who.int/nutrition/publications/micronutrients/guideli nes/calcium_supplementation/en/)

60. WHO recommendations on antenatal care for a positive pregnancy experience. Geneva: World Health Organization; 2016 (http://www.who.int/reproductivehealth/publications/maternal_per inatal_health/anc-positive-pregnancy-experience/en/)

61. The American Heart Association. http://www.goredforwomen.com; Accessed July 12, 2017

62. The Women's Heart Foundation. http://www.womensheart.org. Women's Heart Disease Risk Quiz; Accessed July 12, 2017

INDEX